Liana Goode

Prepari

# Preparing for Pregnancy

Philip J. Robarts
MB, ChB, MRCOG

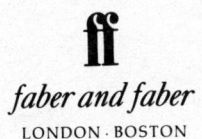

faber and faber
LONDON · BOSTON

First published in 1988
by Faber and Faber Limited
3 Queen Square London WC1N 3AU

Phototypeset by Wilmaset Birkenhead Wirral
Printed in Great Britain by
Richard Clay Ltd Bungay Suffolk
All rights reserved

© Philip J. Robarts, 1988

*This book is sold subject to the condition that it shall not,
by way of trade or otherwise, be lent, resold, hired out
or otherwise circulated without the publisher's prior consent
in any form of binding or cover other than that in which
it is published and without a similar condition including this
condition being imposed on the subsequent purchaser.*

*British Library Cataloguing in Publication Data*

Robarts, Philip J.
Preparing for pregnancy. —— (Popular
medical series).
1. Pregnant women —— Health and hygiene
I. Title II. Series
618.2'4    RG525

ISBN 0–571–15106–X

# Contents

|  | List of illustrations and tables | viii |
|---|---|---|
|  | Author's preface | ix |
|  | Acknowledgements | xi |
| 1 | Introduction | 1 |
| 2 | Reproduction and fetal development | 5 |
| 3 | Contraception | 13 |
| 4 | Diet and nutrition | 17 |
| 5 | Tobacco and alcohol | 27 |
| 6 | Drugs and irradiation | 33 |
| 7 | Infections and pregnancy | 40 |
| 8 | Medical history | 45 |
| 9 | Infertility | 48 |
| 10 | Genetic considerations | 56 |
| 11 | Previous obstetric experience | 63 |
| 12 | Sexual problems | 69 |
| 13 | The early weeks | 73 |
| 14 | Conclusion | 76 |
|  | Glossary | 77 |
|  | Index | 81 |

# Illustrations

| | | |
|---|---|---|
| 2.1. | Control of menstruation | 6 |
| 2.2. | Menstruation and ovulation (schematic description) | 7 |
| 9.1. | Temperature chart demonstrating ovulation | 51 |
| 10.1. | How a baby's sex is determined | 58 |

**Tables**

| | | |
|---|---|---|
| 2.1. | Events leading to menstruation | 8 |
| 2.2. | Developmental times of the fetus in weeks | 10 |
| 2.3. | External characteristics of the fetus | 11 |
| 4.1. | Quetelet index | 19 |
| 4.2. | The three essential nutrients | 21 |
| 7.1. | Risk to fetus from rubella infection in pregnancy | 41 |
| 9.1. | Causes of infertility | 49 |
| 9.2. | Investigations of infertility | 50 |
| 10.1. | Chromosome distribution | 57 |
| 10.2. | Risk of Down's syndrome related to age of mother | 60 |
| 11.1. | Causes of miscarriage | 64 |
| 11.2. | Predisposing factors of tubal pregnancy | 66 |

# Author's Preface

This short book is an attempt to cover those areas which I see as important for people to be aware of when contemplating pregnancy. It has been my deliberate aim to maintain a simple attitude towards the topic rather than for it to develop into a medical textbook and I can only hope that it might prove of some value.

# Acknowledgements

I am indebted to Sheena Glenister for her typing of the manuscript for this book. I should also like to thank Miss P. Downie and Dr E. Forsythe for their help and advice.

# 1
# Introduction

A normal pregnancy, labour and delivery of a healthy, normal baby must be every couple's wish. However, few at some stage do not consider the possibility that their baby might be abnormal. Medical research has introduced many new methods of detecting fetal abnormality and these will be mentioned later. It seems logical, however, to pursue avenues that may minimize the risk of the abnormal occurring and maximize the chance of a normal pregnancy and the subsequent arrival of a healthy baby. It is to these ends that preconceptual or pre-pregnancy care is directed.

With the introduction to this country of the combined oral contraceptive pill (the pill), a simple and effective method of family planning became available. Over the past 20 years, the average size of families has declined and the age of first-time mothers has increased. All the more important, therefore, to consider pre-pregnancy factors that might influence the course of a future pregnancy.

## Improvements in living standards

It is always a tragic occurrence when an infant is stillborn or dies soon after birth. Fortunately, over the years we have seen a steady decline in the number of babies lost, thanks to improvements in general living conditions and standards, and obstetric care. This decline can best be illustrated by looking at the change that has occurred in the perinatal mortality rate. This is calculated from the number of stillborn

## Introduction

infants and babies dying during the first week of life and dividing this figure by the total numbers of infants delivered. It is expressed as a rate per thousand for individual hospitals, district and regional health authorities, and nationally.

For example, the perinatal mortality rate for England and Wales in the early 1950s was around 38, whereas in 1984 this figure had dropped to approximately eleven.

There are obvious reasons for this improvement. General living conditions and standards have improved, as has obstetric care itself with the advent of routine screening procedures for the detection of fetal abnormalities.

How much lower can we hope to see this figure drop? However vigilant the care of pregnant women is, during both the antenatal period and labour, two factors still provide a significant contribution to the perinatal mortality figures – premature birth and congenital abnormality of the baby.

**Prematurity**

One of the mysteries of obstetrics still remaining is the mechanism by which the onset of labour is determined. We know of many situations which predispose to premature onset, and drugs have been developed to attempt to suppress the uterus contracting. The main advance in the reduction of fetal loss from this cause is the dramatic improvement in the skills of those who care for the very low birth-weight infant.

**Fetal abnormalities**

Approximately 2 per cent of all infants have a significant abnormality. In half of these the defects are such that stillbirth or death during the first year of life results. In the remainder, specialized help is needed to reduce the severity of the handicap or merely to sustain life. Although the obstetrician is frequently called upon to inform parents of an

## Introduction

abnormal newborn child it must be appreciated that only about 50 per cent of defects noted during the first year of life are detected at delivery.

### CHROMOSOME ABNORMALITIES

Abnormalities of the chromosomes, a disturbance in the genetic make-up of the baby, occur about 6 every 1000 deliveries. In certain situations, such as the older pregnant woman or a strong family history of a genetic illness, tests such as amniocentesis or chorionic villus sampling (see Chapter 10) can be undertaken to exclude an abnormality in early pregnancy. Many abnormalities, however, occur sporadically, without warning, so cannot be detected before birth.

### OTHER CAUSES

Other recognized causes of fetal abnormality are ionizing radiation (for example, X-rays), infections during pregnancy, drugs and – less well recognized, although becoming increasingly investigated – nutritional deficiency. It must be said at the outset, however, that in the vast majority of cases where an abnormal baby is born no identifiable cause can be found. Similarly, the causes of miscarriage and premature labour remain poorly understood.

## The preconception clinic

In the following chapters, I shall try and define certain aspects of health care which are pertinent to the issue of preconceptual care. For many people, most of this will be nothing new. The hazards of smoking and alcohol and the benefits of an adequate diet are well known, although in this book these areas are discussed in the specific context of pre-pregnancy planning and their possible effects on pregnancy itself.

Apart from general health measures, problems arising from previous pregnancies have to be considered. Couples, understandably, are interested in knowing the likelihood of prob-

## Introduction

lems recurring and this is the area of pre-conceptual care. So where is such help to be obtained? One's family doctor or a member of his team such as the health visitor are obvious sources, but sometimes referral to specialists such as obstetricians or geneticists may be necessary. An optimal solution is in the preconception or pregnancy planning clinic where advice can be given and information sought with direct recourse to help in specific situations.

Preconception clinics are becoming increasingly common as this field of medicine gains wider acceptance of its importance but this type of care and advice does not guarantee a normal pregnancy and baby. What I hope this book may achieve is to stimulate an awareness that there are opportunities of improving the likelihood of this goal by simply altering one's habits or seeking medical advice before embarking on a pregnancy.

# 2
# Reproduction and fetal development

If consideration is to be given to factors important in preconceptual care, it is important first to grasp the mechanisms that control production of the egg and the sperm, together with the events that occur during the early stages of development of the unborn child.

**The menstrual cycle**

Let us first consider the events that occur during each menstrual cycle. The average length of cycle is 28 days, the most important feature being the production of an egg or ovum. Figures 2.1 and 2.2 are a simplified representation of what happens and can be summarized as follows:

1. A part of the brain called the hypothalamus produces hormones (chemical messengers) which act on the pituitary gland, a tiny structure lying at the base of the brain.

2. Under this stimulation, the pituitary gland produces two hormones:
    (a) follicle stimulating hormone (FSH), and
    (b) luteinizing hormone (LH).

3. These hormones then act upon the ovary, which contains numerous follicles, small cysts containing the egg cells. Each month, one of these follicles enlarges under the influence of FSH, ruptures and releases an ovum – as a result of a surge of LH – ovulation has occurred.

# Reproduction and fetal development

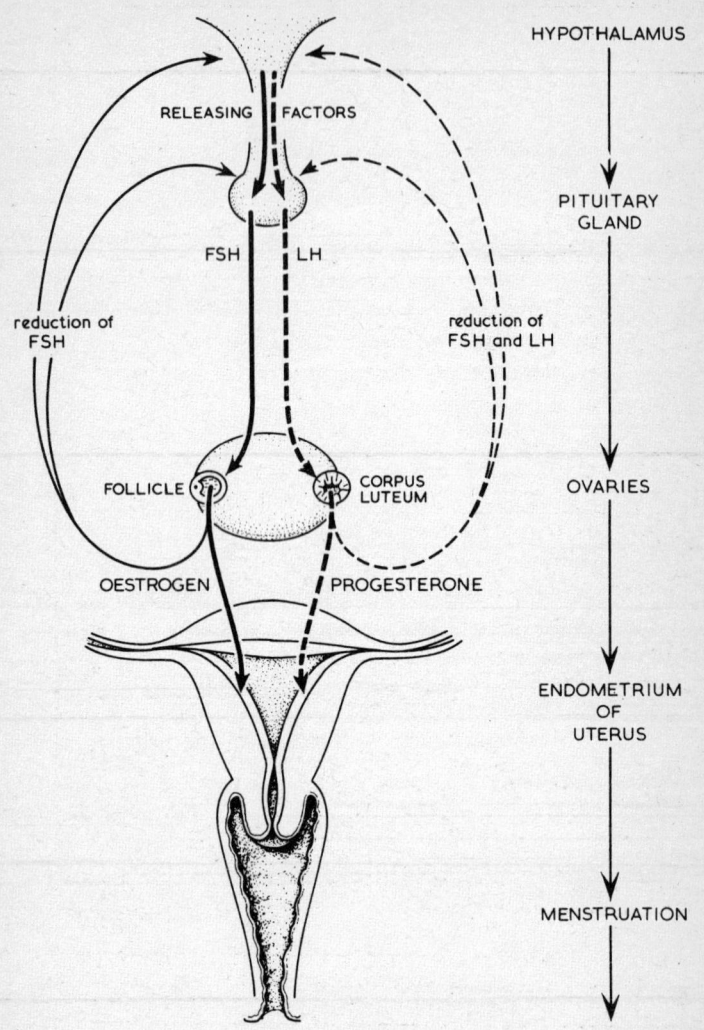

Figure 2.1 Control of menstruation

## Reproduction and fetal development

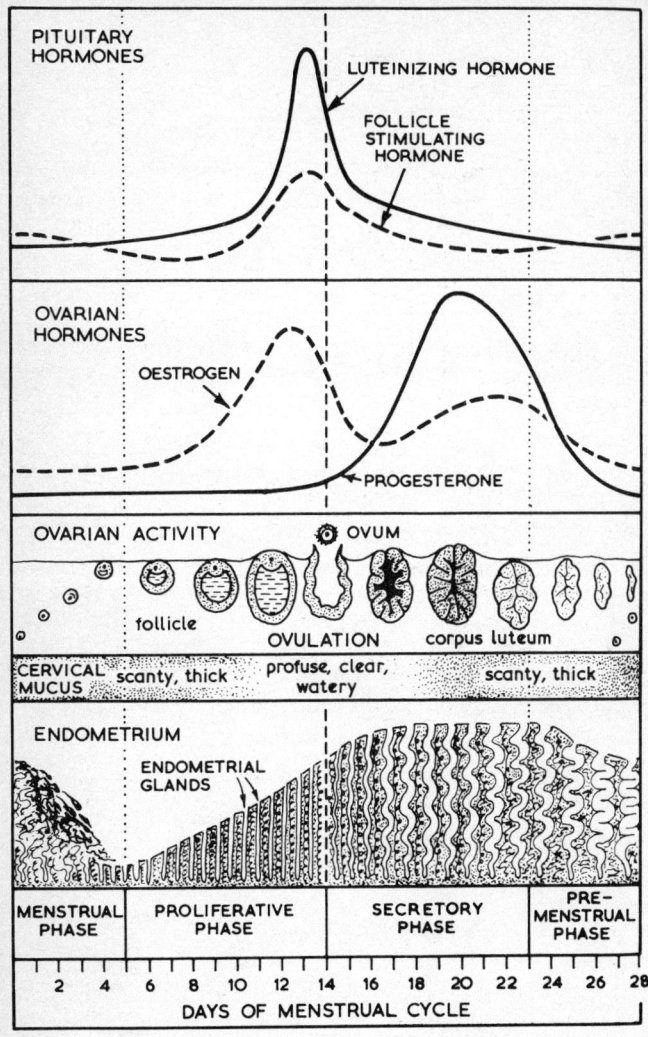

Figure 2.2 Menstruation and ovulation (schematic description)

4. During enlargement of the follicle the hormone oestrogen is produced. Following ovulation the follicle collapses and is then called a corpus luteum ('yellow body'). This produces the hormone progesterone.

5. Oestrogen and progesterone have important effects on the lining of the womb (the endometrium). Oestrogen produces thickening or proliferation of the endometrium before progesterone acts to fill the glands in the endometrium with secretions in preparation for implantation of the egg should fertilization take place.

6. If fertilization does not occur then the corpus luteum degenerates, oestrogen and progesterone levels fall and the endometrium is shed, appearing as blood; this is called menstruation.

This complex series of events is summarized in Table 2.1.

**Table 2.1** Events leading to menstruation

|  | *Number of days* |
|---|---|
| 1. After menstruation a follicle ripens: oestrogen is produced: the endometrium proliferates | 10 |
| 2. Ovulation | |
| 3. The corpus luteum appears: progesterone is produced: small amounts of oestrogen persist: the endometrium becomes secretory | 14 |
| 4. The corpus luteum degenerates: oestrogen and progesterone levels fall: menstruation | 4 |
| Total | 28 |

## Reproduction and fetal development

### Sperm production

Spermatogenesis, the production of sperm, although less readily recognizable is, like the menstrual cycle, a delicate process no less subject to disturbance than ovulation.

Sperm production occurs in the tubules of the testes under the influence of FSH and of testosterone, formed in the testes by the stimulus of LH. Secretion of these hormones is virtually continuous following the onset of puberty. The formation of a mature sperm is a process involving several stages, at the end of which it may survive for several weeks within the male reproductive tract.

Because the whole business is reliant on the production of hormones by the hypothalamus and anterior pituitary gland, it may well be disrupted by external factors such as stress, smoking or excessive alcohol intake. Infections such as mumps can also have an adverse effect on sperm production.

Analysis of a normal sample of semen should reveal more than 40 million sperm per millilitre (ml), 75 per cent of which should be normally formed, and over 50 per cent of which should be motile.

### Conception

For conception to occur a sperm must penetrate an ovum. The sequence of events leading up to this is as follows:

1. The end of a healthy Fallopian tube, which hangs over the ovary, consists of finger-like processes (fimbriae), which pick up the released ovum. This is then wafted down the tube by the hair-like processes (cilia) that line the surface of the tube. An egg has a life of about 24–36 hours.

2. During intercourse, ejaculation results in millions of sperm being deposited in the upper vagina and around the cervix. The cervical mucus around the time of ovulation is

## Reproduction and fetal development

highly amenable to sperm penetration. Only a few hundred thousand sperm reach the cavity of the uterus, however, and only a few thousand enter the Fallopian tubes. Ultimately, of course, only one sperm penetrates the centre of the ovum and fuses with the female nucleus – conception has occurred.

3. The fertilized egg continues its journey towards the cavity of the uterus and forms itself into a tiny ball of cells, known as a morula. This reaches the cavity of the uterus 5–7 days following fertilization and embeds itself in the lining, being fully implanted by day 28 of the menstrual cycle.

4. The endometrium, already thickened during the second (secretory) half of the cycle, now becomes even further developed, with a rich blood supply, and is known as the decidua.

5. Once the morula reaches the uterus it develops a central cavity and is called a blastocyst. This comprises an outer shell of cells which will ultimately form the placenta, and an inner

**Table 2.2** Developmental times of the fetus in weeks

|  | *Differentiation* | *Complete formation* |
| --- | --- | --- |
| Spinal cord | 3–4 | 20 |
| Brain | 3 | 28 |
| Eyes | 3 | 20–24 |
| Ears | 3–4 | 24–28 |
| Lungs | 5 | 24–28 |
| Heart | 3 | 6 |
| Intestinal system | 3 | 24 |
| Kidneys | 3–4 | 12 |
| Genital organs | 5 | 7 |
| Face | 3–4 | 8 |
| Limbs | 4–5 | 8 |

## Reproduction and fetal development

**Table 2.3** External characteristics of the fetus

| Period of gestation (in weeks from last menstrual period) | Length of fetus (Crown–rump length, cm) | Characteristics |
|---|---|---|
| 8 | 2.5 | Nose, external ears, fingers, toes are identifiable but featureless. Head is fixed on thorax |
| 12 | 9.0 | External ears show main features, eyelids fused, neck has formed and external genitals formed but undifferentiated |
| 16 | 18.0 | External genitals can be differentiated, skin is transparent red |
| 20 | 25.0 | Skin becoming opaque, fine hair covers body |
| 24 | 32.0 | Eyelids separated, eyebrows and eyelashes present, skin wrinkled |

mound of cells, the inner cell mass, from which the embryo will develop.

As the placenta develops it takes over production of progesterone and oestrogen from the corpus luteum, which regresses after 10–12 weeks.

### Fetal development

The development of the fetus falls into three stages. The first stage, described above, is from fertilization to successful

## Reproduction and fetal development

implantation. The second stage is from then until the end of the 8th week, by which time the development of nearly all the major organs has begun and the embryo begins to look recognizably human. The third stage, from the 8th week until delivery, is largely one of organ growth and development.

The times at which the various organs begin to develop (differentiate) and are completely formed are shown in Table 2.2. Table 2.3 shows the size and external appearance of the fetus at various gestational ages.

This then is a highly simplified description of how the fetus grows from a single fertilized cell into a complex organism, increasing its weight during the process by about six billion times.

# 3
# Contraception

We are now fortunate to have great control over when and how many children we have. The widespread use of effective forms of contraception such as the combined oral contraceptive pill and the intrauterine contraceptive device (IUCD) have helped make this possible, although it is disappointing to note the continuously rising rate in the number of pregnancies ending in therapeutic abortion (termination).

In preconceptual care, the questions pertaining to contraception revolve around: how long to discontinue the method prior to embarking on pregnancy; and equally important, what risks are involved should conception occur while the contraceptive method of choice is still in use, for no form of contraception is 100 per cent effective.

Barrier methods of contraception such as the sheath and diaphragm provide relatively few problems in terms of complications. However, the pill and the coil have both attracted much attention over the years, particularly in association with fetal abnormality. Below I shall consider more closely both the combined oral contraceptive pill and the progesterone-only pill, and the intrauterine contraceptive device in planning a pregnancy.

**The combined pill**

This is a mixture of the hormones oestrogen and progesterone, usually as synthetic derivatives. It was first introduced into this country in the early 1960s and is a highly effective form of contraception. Like any other drug, however, it has its recognized side-effects, although sophistication in its exact composition has reduced these over the years.

The contraceptive effect is achieved by preventing ovulation through inhibition of the LH surge (see Chapter 2). There is also alteration in the cervical mucus rendering it relatively hostile to sperm. There had been much speculation regarding the possibility of the pill having a harmful effect on future pregnancies, such as a higher rate of miscarriage or fetal abnormalities.

A large study was therefore set up in the late 1960s and reported in the medical literature in 1976 by the Royal College of General Practitioners.* They looked at the outcome of some 15 000 pregnancies among former oral contraceptive pill-users and a control group who had never taken the pill. They reported no difference in the miscarriage rate between the two groups and no evidence of any harmful effects of the pill on subsequent fetal outcome.

Much has been written regarding the possible harmful effects of the combined pill on the fetus if taken inadvertently during pregnancy. A wide variety of abnormalities have been reported, however, and it seems unlikely that their cause can be related to one particular factor.

In general, I would recommend the pill be discontinued 3 to 6 months prior to starting a pregnancy, so that a regular menstrual cycle may be re-established. Barrier methods of contraception may be used during this time, so one can be much more certain about the date of the last menstrual period and the calculation of the expected date of delivery.

* 'The outcome of pregnancy in former oral contraceptive users', Royal College of General Practitioners' Oral Contraception Study Group, *British Journal of Obstetrics and Gynaecology*, August 1976, Vol. 83, pp. 608–16.

## Contraception

### Progesterone-only pill

The so-called mini-pill contains only a progesterone derivative, with no oestrogen component. Although it may have some action in suppressing ovulation, its main role is in the alteration of the cervical mucus and the motility of the tubes and uterus, thus impairing fertilization and implantation.

### Intrauterine contraceptive device

The IUCD or coil is not as effective a form of contraception as oral contraceptives but it does have several advantages: its effects are confined to the reproductive organs, and it obviates the need for daily pill-taking which many women find a nuisance.

Numerous types have evolved over the years. Initially, these were all plastic forms, but today most also contain a copper wire wound around the stem which seems to improve their efficiency. The exact mode of contraceptive effect, however, is still poorly understood, although it seems most likely that a local reaction in the lining of the womb caused by the presence of the coil prevents implantation of the embryo. It is not clear whether the coil has any effect on the process of fertilization. Upon its removal the reaction within the womb quickly dies down, and as with the pill one would advise waiting around 3 to 6 months before embarking on a pregnancy.

The coil is approximately 98 per cent effective at preventing pregnancy. But there is a recognized association between the coil and tubal pregnancy – the embryo implanting in the lining of the Fallopian tube instead of the womb. Should one become pregnant with a coil *in situ*, medical advice should be sought at an early stage to confirm the site of the pregnancy.

Other risks are associated with pregnancy and the coil, in

## Contraception

particular a greater risk of miscarriage or premature labour later in pregnancy. I favour removal of the coil in early pregnancy if at all possible. Fortunately, there seems to be no increase in the abnormality rate of babies resulting from these pregnancies even when the copper devices are involved.

# 4

# Diet and nutrition

Fortunately, in this country today severe nutritional deficiency is rare. Indeed, a far greater problem lies in the mildly or grossly obese. Extremes of body weight have serious implications in terms of a woman conceiving. As we have seen earlier in this book, the mechanisms that control ovulation are highly complex and sensitive. The woman who suffers from anorexia nervosa, with a greatly reduced body weight, characteristically no longer has regular menstrual periods, often none at all (amenorrhoea), as ovulation ceases to occur. On the other hand, the grossly obese woman may also often complain of irregular periods, through loss of normal ovary function. When treating women with such menstrual disturbances, whether associated with impaired fertility or not, it is important to enquire into recent changes in weight, as restoring normal body weight often restores regular menstruation and fertility.

## Nutrition

FOOD DEPRIVATION

The importance of adequate nutrition during pregnancy and around the time of conception has been well illustrated by looking at instances of severe food deprivation. The best documented are famines that occurred during the Second World War. During the seige of Leningrad, which lasted for almost 18 months, thousands of people died from starvation. The average birth weight of babies born during this period

## Diet and nutrition

fell by around 500 g and half of those weighed less than 2.5 kg at birth.

During the winter of 1944, famine affected cities in western Holland over a period of 6 months (the Dutch Hunger Winter). Adequate food supplies were available before and after this spell, so pregnant women were not exposed to this problem for the whole duration of pregnancy. Those suffering nutritional deprivation over the last few months of pregnancy gave birth to underweight babies, while those who had eaten adequately during the latter stage of pregnancy delivered infants of normal birth weight.

This illustrates the fact that these final weeks of pregnancy are important in terms of fetal growth; indeed one would expect that under normal circumstances the fetus would treble its weight over the final 12 weeks of pregnancy.

### EARLY PREGNANCY

So much for the importance of nutrition during pregnancy – what about its significance in very early pregnancy and around the time of conception? One of the striking features of the famines described above was the marked rise in the incidence of amenorrhoea in women in the reproductive age group, which seemed directly related to lack of food. During the latter months of the Dutch famine the conception rate fell to half of that prior to food shortage, and further examination suggested that malnutrition around the time of conception might be significant in causing congenital abnormalities. We have seen in Chapter 2 how most of the major organ systems are beginning to develop during the first 8 weeks of pregnancy and it is reasonable to speculate that abnormalities of the baby might stem from some dietary omission during these early stages. It was noted particularly that the increase in premature births and the infant mortality rate associated with the Dutch famine was not among those born *during* this food shortage but among those who had

## Diet and nutrition

been conceived during the famine and were born some months later.

### IDEAL HEIGHT AND WEIGHT

Apart from these extreme circumstances – what is the ideal weight and ideal diet to be aimed for prior to conception?

Numerous tables are available giving ideal body weights in relation to height, stature, age etc. Another useful measure is known as the Quetelet index (Table 4.1). This is calculated by the formula $W/H^2$–weight (W) in kilograms (kg), divided by height (H) squared where height is in metres (m). Height and weight are measured in indoor clothes but without shoes, giving a figure from which one can judge one's own weight. Table 4.1 shows examples for a woman of 1.62 m (5' 4"), and with the aid of a pocket calculator one can calculate one's own Quetelet index.

**Table 4.1** Quetelet index

| $\dfrac{\text{Weight in kg}}{(\text{height in metres})^2}$ | for example, | $\dfrac{58.5}{1.62 \times 1.62} = 22.3$ |
|---|---|---|

| Quetelet index | | Typical weight |
|---|---|---|
| less than 20 | underweight | 50 kg (8 st 1 lb) |
| 20–25 | ideal | 58 kg (9 st 3 lb) |
| 26–30 | moderately overweight | 71.5 kg (11 st 5 lb) |
| greater than 30 | grossly obese | 78 kg (12 st 7 lb) |

### Diet

There are four major chemical components to the food we eat: carbohydrates, fats, proteins, and minerals and vitamins. One must also remember the essential role of water and salts. Let us briefly look at these nutrients and the role they play.

## Diet and nutrition

### CARBOHYDRATES

Carbohydrates provide the main source of energy in most diets and the commoner types are starch, cellulose and sugar. Starch and cellulose are composed of hundreds of sugar molecules joined together in a chain. While starch is a principal energy source for humans, cellulose (a major component of vegetable matter) cannot be absorbed or utilized by man. Sugar comes in various forms – sucrose is the alternative name for table sugar, while lactose is the sugar found in milk and dairy produce.

### FATS

Fats are the next most important energy source and a more concentrated form of energy than carbohydrates. Some forms of fats are known as 'essential' fatty acids, which the human body cannot manufacture itself. They are also called polyunsaturated fatty acids and have gained much publicity from the finding that they lower cholesterol levels in the blood and protect against diseases such as heart attacks.

### PROTEINS

Proteins form the very structure of human tissues and are therefore a vital dietary constituent to replace the continuous breakdown of body proteins. During times of rapid growth such as pregnancy and childhood, increased amounts of protein are required in the diet.

In Table 4.2 are listed some of the commoner foods that contain these three essential nutrients – carbohydrates, fats and proteins.

The secret of formulating an adequate diet lies in balancing the intake of nutrients together with providing some variety in the form they take. Equally important is that, having chosen the appropriate foods, their nutritional value is not diminished by improper preparation, this is of particular importance with regard to vitamins, a rich source of which is derived from fruit and vegetables.

*Diet and nutrition*

**Table 4.2** The three essential nutrients

| Proteins | Fats | Carbohydrates |
| --- | --- | --- |
| Meat | Dairy products | Cereals |
| Fish | Meat | Pasta |
| Cheese | Margarine | Pulses, lentils etc. |
| Milk, etc. | Oils | Flour |
| Eggs | | Sugar |
| Dried beans and peas | | Dried fruit |
| Pasta | | Potatoes |
| Cereals (including rice) | | |

VITAMINS

Vitamins are chemical substances which the body is unable to manufacture itself. They must be supplied in the diet and various specific vitamin deficiency states are now well recognized. Equally well recognized is that vitamin deficiency in the maternal diet during pregnancy can lead to offspring being born with vitamin deficiency conditions.

Vitamins can be divided into two classes – those soluble in fat, and those soluble in water. The body cannot maintain a large store of water-soluble vitamins as they are eliminated readily through the kidneys. In contrast, the fat-soluble vitamins are stored in large amounts in the liver. So vitamin deficiency of water-soluble varieties may arise over a matter of weeks of inadequate dietary intake, while months or years may elapse before the fat-soluble vitamin deficiency state becomes manifest.

*Vitamin A*

This is a fat-soluble vitamin with large stores in the liver, so deficiency is most unlikely in the western world. Indeed, it has been shown that excessive doses of vitamin A taken in early pregnancy can produce abnormalities of the fetal skull

## Diet and nutrition

and facial bones, so excessive use of capsules from health food manufacturers are to be avoided. There is little danger of reaching toxic levels other than through medication.

Vitamin A is important in the development of bones and teeth and also plays an important role in normal vision. Major sources of the vitamin lie in dairy products, liver and in particular oils such as cod-liver oil which is exceptionally rich. Carrots, spinach and tomatoes are also good sources.

### Vitamin B complex

Vitamin B has a number of types, all with a specific function to perform. Thiamine, riboflavine, nicotinic acid and folic acid are all B vitamins. Red meat, yeast, pulses, rice and vegetables such as broccoli, sprouts and spinach all contain vitamins from the B group. Folic acid can also be obtained from oranges and bananas and is of particular importance in the prevention of anaemia, as is vitamin $B_{12}$.

### Vitamin C

Vitamin C, or ascorbic acid, is a water-soluble vitamin, deficiency of which results in the condition called scurvy. Fresh fruit and vegetables provide a rich source of the vitamin, but it is easily destroyed by heating, so cooking can dramatically reduce the amount available. It is important in binding cells together, promoting healing and preventing anaemia.

### Vitamin D

This is a fat-soluble vitamin and is stored in the liver. Deficiency gives rise to the condition known as rickets with twisting of the leg bones and the spine. This is an unusual condition today, but serves as a reminder of the importance of the vitamin in forming and hardening bones. Food sources of the vitamin are fish-liver oils, butter, milk, cheese and eggs, and liver itself. It can also be manufactured in the fat lying under the skin by the action of ultraviolet light, and

## Diet and nutrition

explains the incidence of rickets in the past among children living in industrial cities who had little exposure to sunlight.

A balanced diet should provide all the necessary vitamins. It has long been known from experiments with animals that deficiency of vitamins in the mother's diet in pregnancy can cause the offspring to be born with vitamin deficiency diseases and that both deficiency and excess of vitamins can cause a wide range of developmental abnormalities in the newborn.

### MINERALS AND TRACE ELEMENTS

Before considering the question of vitamin supplements, we should also discuss certain minerals and trace elements that play an equally important part in our diet.

Certain simple elements such as iron and zinc are, like vitamins, essential in the complex processes of human function and fetal development. We also know of the harmful effects of other elements such as lead, cadmium and mercury.

### *Iron*

Most pregnant women take iron tablets during their pregnancy, though actually, provided there is no iron deficiency prior to pregnancy and a normal diet is consumed, there is probably no real need as iron absorption increases throughout pregnancy to compensate for the increased requirements. The rationale for giving all pregnant women iron supplements is that it is simpler than attempting to identify individual women who may be iron-deficient.

### *Zinc*

It is now possible to measure levels of many substances in the human body, and one which may play an important part in normal fetal development is zinc. Zinc is known as an essential trace element and we know that it is involved in many vital chemical processes such as protein formation.

## Diet and nutrition

Once again, animal studies suggest that zinc deficiency in the mother can lead to impairment of intelligence in the offspring. Neural depression, including postnatal depression, may be a symptom of zinc deficiency and the increased amounts of zinc lost in the urine of alcoholics may be partly responsible for the fetal alcohol syndrome (see Chapter 5).

As mentioned earlier, vitamin deficiency may also be involved in the causation of spina bifida and related disorders, as zinc is required for the absorption of some of these vitamins from the gut.

So zinc is obviously an important element in one's diet. A survey in 1981 produced by the Ministry of Agriculture, Fisheries and Food (MAFF) suggested that the typical daily diet contained only half the necessary amount of zinc and probably less for vegetarians. So should zinc tablets be taken? It appears that there is mounting evidence to suggest the benefits of zinc supplementation before, during and after pregnancy, but we must wait for official confirmation.

### Iodine
Iodine deficiency in the mother is well known to lead to cretinism in her offspring, a severe form of mental retardation.

### Cadmium, mercury, lead
Excessive amounts of the elements cadmium, mercury and lead have also been found to be associated with an increased incidence of fetal abnormalities, impairment of fetal growth and even fetal death.

So how does one know one's status in terms of these trace elements? The answer is not simple – hair analysis has been widely suggested as a method, but it is far from accurate and results can be misleading. Analysis of blood is probably the simplest means but this too has inaccuracies and the tests are not widely available. However, by adopting a balanced diet

## Diet and nutrition

with adequate variety all the trace elements should be obtained without resorting to supplementation.

SUPPLEMENTATION

The use of iron supplementation in the treatment and prevention of anaemia is often combined with folic acid which also plays a role in red blood cell production.

In 1933, there was shown to be a link between vitamin A deficiency and birth defects in piglets – notably absence of the eyes. Then, in 1941 bone abnormalities in the offspring of rats were shown to be due to deficient diets. Since the mid-1960s, speculation has surrounded the possibility that deficiency of vitamins might have a part to play in the cause of spina bifida and related abnormalities of the central nervous system in human infants.

Neural tube defects, of which spina bifida is one type, are developmental abnormalities of the central nervous system, affecting either the brain itself, the spinal cord, or both. There are probably numerous factors involved in its occurrence, but it is most common among infants born to women in the lower social classes. This led researchers to surmise that there might be more likelihood of their diet being deficient in some specific factor. So a trial was set up in which women who had had a previously affected infant were offered vitamin supplementation prior to and during their subsequent pregnancy. The final analysis is yet to be announced, but preliminary results suggest that despite all the other associated factors that might be implicated, vitamin supplementation appears to play an important part in a low recurrence rate.

Specific vitamin deficiency states are well recognized in infants of mothers who have an inadequate diet in vitamins. So why shouldn't vitamin supplementation be offered to all pregnant women? Unfortunately, this solution is not quite as simple as it may seem, for while diseases may be caused by

## Diet and nutrition

vitamin deficiency, it is also recognized that excessive amounts of vitamins taken by pregnant women may cause abnormalities – excessive vitamin A, for example, is known to be associated with facial abnormalities such as hare lip and cleft palate. Until further evidence is available, therefore, it would appear wise to confine oneself to an adequate diet rather than resort to vitamin supplementation unless under specific medical direction.

So one's diet and weight are very important factors in pre-pregnancy planning. It is also worth remembering that some form of regular exercise is of equal benefit not only prior to and during pregnancy but throughout one's life.

The amount and type of exercise undertaken will vary, of course, from person to person, and will also depend on their occupation. Activities such as squash can be extremely vigorous and it is important to develop exercise tolerance gradually. Whatever one's pursuit, be it jogging, swimming, aerobics or other sports, the more often it is undertaken, the fitter one will become.

People with certain medical conditions may be well advised, however, to ask their doctor for his advice before undertaking increased amounts of exercise.

# 5

# Tobacco and alcohol

**Smoking**

Even the most dedicated smoker cannot deny that smoking is bad for one's health in general terms, and if contemplating pregnancy she must now accept that smoking constitutes a very real hazard to the outcome of the pregnancy. As long ago as 1935 it was noted that the fetal heart rate increased shortly after a mother began to smoke a cigarette. It was suggested that this was caused by a toxic agent, such as nicotine, crossing the placenta and affecting the fetus. Studies suggest that smoking could account for 30 per cent of all low birth-weight babies and up to 10 per cent of perinatal deaths (stillbirths and babies dying during the first week of life).

ADVERSE EFFECTS ON HEALTH

The adverse effects of smoking may be related to increased levels of nicotine, carbon monoxide or cyanide, or a combination of these and other harmful chemicals which enter the blood-stream of smokers or those who are exposed to tobacco smoke from nearby smokers. The effects of smoking are dependent on the numbers of cigarettes smoked, and seem more pronounced in older women and those already with chest conditions.

The problems in general health terms associated with smoking such as lung cancer, bronchitis and heart disease are well recognized. Suffice to say that, depending on the number of cigarettes smoked, there is up to a five-fold increase in lung cancer among women who smoke; by stopping smoking the

## Tobacco and alcohol

risk can be gradually decreased to that of a non-smoker over a period of 15 years. Women under the age of fifty who smoke in excess of 40 cigarettes a day have a 20 times greater risk of a heart attack compared to non-smokers. The incidence of strokes is also increased by smoking.

At one time it was thought that women were relatively protected from the effects of smoking on blood vessel disease, but studies now suggest that the risk from smoking is as great in women as in men. Increasing age and the use of the combined oral contraceptive pill seem to be major factors in raising the risk of cardiovascular disease from smoking.

A recent survey in the United States suggested that approximately 30 per cent of women were smokers when they conceived. The majority smoked less than 20 cigarettes a day. About a quarter stopped smoking during pregnancy, and a further third drastically reduced the number they smoked.

### EFFECTS ON THE PREGNANT MOTHER

So what effects does smoking have on the pregnant mother? Apart from the fetal problem of decreased birth weight, some studies have suggested an increased incidence of bleeding from the afterbirth during the latter stages of pregnancy. The bleeding can arise from both the afterbirth lying low in the womb (placenta praevia), and also from it partially separating from the wall of the womb prematurely (placental abruption).

Another side-effect attributed to smoking is that of poor weight gain by the mother during pregnancy. It is probably true that people often eat more and gain weight having stopped smoking, but the reverse – that pregnant women who smoke eat less – is not always the case. Calculations based on the calorie intake of pregnant women, smokers and non- smokers, suggest that smoking increases the body's metabolic rate, the rate at which energy stores are used,

## Tobacco and alcohol

leading to a reduced weight gain, reflected in the reduced fetal weight among mothers who smoke.

### EFFECTS ON THE UNBORN BABY

How does smoking affect the unborn baby? Over the last 25 years, numerous articles in the medical press have led to the conclusion that babies of smokers weigh 150 to 200 g less than non-smokers' babies, and twice as many babies will weigh less than 2.5 kg if the mother smokes. These weight differences seem to be directly related to the number of cigarettes smoked. The risk, of course, is also influenced by a number of other factors such as age, height and pre-pregnancy weight. Even having corrected for these variations, women who smoke less than 20 cigarettes a day increase the risk of perinatal loss by 20 per cent, and those who smoke more than this increase the risk by up to 35 per cent over that of non-smokers. This increased perinatal mortality rate seems to be due largely to premature delivery.

The incidence of miscarriage and abnormal babies seems to be increased among smokers, directly related to the number of cigarettes smoked. It has also been suggested that infants of mothers who smoked during pregnancy have impaired intellectual development, and that hyperactive children are also commoner.

### EFFECTS ON MEN

The focus so far has been directed on the effects of smoking on mother and unborn child. In men, however, quite apart from the risks of heart and lung disease, smoking impairs sperm production, not only in terms of numbers of sperm but also their morphology and motility, which may contribute to the increased miscarriage and fetal abnormality rates. The prospect of pregnancy, therefore, creates the ideal opportunity for both partners to stop smoking and they should give one another every encouragement to do so.

## Alcohol

It is now well established that alcohol consumed during pregnancy can cause harm to the fetus. This can range from precipitating miscarriage to a recognized group of abnormalities known as the 'fetal alcohol syndrome'.

HISTORICAL BACKGROUND

A connection between alcohol and fetal abnormality was first suspected during the eighteenth century. In 1759, the Royal College of Physicians in London requested Parliament to reinstate taxation on gin to render it less affordable and consequently reduce the risk of exposing the fetus to it. Parliament ultimately complied with this request, and has continued to do so ever since! However, the warnings regarding drinking during pregnancy continued to be given, suggesting that the problem persisted despite the change in the law.

In 1899 came the first published evidence of the adverse effects of alcohol during pregnancy. A Dr Sullivan compared 600 offspring of 120 alcoholic women imprisoned in Liverpool jail with offspring born to 28 teetotal female relations of these prisoners. He showed a mortality rate during the first year of life and a stillbirth rate two and a half times that of infants born to the non-alcoholic women. He also demonstrated that alcoholic women who had previously delivered babies with serious abnormalities gave birth to normal infants when forced to abstain from alcohol due to their imprisonment.

Modern recognition of alcohol as an agent harmful to the fetus did not occur until 1973 when two articles were published in *The Lancet* by workers in the Department of Paediatrics in Seattle, USA. They described mental retardation, abnormalities of the face and heart together with developmental delay occurring in eleven children born to alcoholic mothers and coined the phrase 'fetal alcohol syndrome'.

## Tobacco and alcohol

#### FETAL ALCOHOL SYNDROME

The fetal alcohol syndrome has now been described by doctors all over the world. It is not an especially common condition, on a worldwide basis having a prevalence of 1 to 3 cases per 1000 births. Obviously, if one confines the study to alcoholic mothers then the prevalence rises sharply. Indeed, it has been suggested that exposure of the fetus to alcohol accounts for up to 5 per cent of all abnormalities, which represents a significant proportion of previously unexplained abnormalities. If accurate, then alcohol obviously represents a major contribution to abnormal fetal development. Also, in terms of mental retardation, alcohol abuse during pregnancy must now be considered a major cause.

#### OTHER EFFECTS OF ALCOHOL ON PREGNANCY

Before an infant can be said to have the fetal alcohol syndrome a number of criteria must be fulfilled. There are several other conditions, however, which can arise in isolation following alcohol abuse during pregnancy.

The risk of miscarriage is approximately doubled by maternal drinking, though probably only among the heavier drinkers. A lower birth weight is probably the most commonly observed effect of alcohol in pregnancy and seems to be dose-related. Even taking into account other factors such as age, height and smoking, this decrease holds good. Among heavy drinkers, there is certainly an increased risk of premature delivery and growth-retarded infants.

Abnormal behavioural development among these infants has also been recognized, in particular, delay in mental development and an increased incidence of hyperactivity.

#### ALCOHOL ABUSE AND PREGNANCY

It has proved extremely difficult to determine the timing and the amount of alcohol consumption during pregnancy which puts the fetus most at risk. This is largely due to the problem

## Tobacco and alcohol

of obtaining accurate information regarding drinking patterns and the amount consumed. Also, of course, drinking habits often alter as pregnancy progresses.

The commonest question asked about alcohol and pregnancy is whether there is a safe level of alcohol intake and, if so, what is it? Advising abstinence from alcohol for women who are pregnant or contemplating pregnancy is perfectly reasonable but unlikely to be of practical value.

Animal studies, producing low to moderate blood alcohol levels, have shown no fetal effects and the abnormalities discussed so far are among the offspring of very heavy drinkers; indeed, approximately half of their infants will be unaffected in any way. Moderation, therefore, must be the key word.

### PATERNAL DRINKING

It has been suggested that some alcohol-related birth defects could be caused by excessive drinking in the father. Abnormalities of sperm have been noted among male alcoholics which could be responsible for fetal abnormalities. But as yet no convincing evidence has come to light.

### CONCLUSION

We know that alcohol can cause fetal abnormality when consumed to excess. Prevention of alcohol-related birth defects, however, is more likely to come about through tackling the problem of alcohol abuse in general. Small quantities of alcohol consumed in pregnancy seem unlikely to be harmful, but as yet, nobody can stipulate a safe limit.

# 6

# Drugs and irradiation

**Adverse drug effects on the fetus**

Any harm that a drug might cause to the fetus is largely dependent on what stage of the pregnancy it is taken. If this is during the early weeks, the period of organogenesis, when the vital organs are formed, then malformations may be produced. During the middle and later stages of pregnancy any harmful effects of drugs are likely to be in terms of growth and functional development of the fetus. However, we are most concerned with malformations caused by those drugs known as teratogens.

THALIDOMIDE

In 1958, in order to prevent sleepnessness and sickness in the early weeks of pregnancy, the drug thalidomide was prescribed in this country. The ensuing tragedies during 1959 and 1960 clearly demonstrated that drugs prescribed in pregnancy might do no harm, indeed might benefit the mother, but could result in disastrous consequences for the developing embryo. The terrible results of thalidomide also heightened the awareness of both the general public and medical profession alike of the dangers of taking any medicines in early pregnancy.

In retrospect, we now know that 25 per cent of babies born to mothers who had taken thalidomide were affected with serious limb abnormalities. One would like to think that this sort of situation could not arise today with the rigorous testing of drugs and the regulations surrounding their safety.

## Drugs and irradiation

It is interesting to remember that administration of thalidomide to pregnant mice resulted in no abnormalities of the offspring and this highlights the problem of trying to extrapolate to humans from animal experimentation.

### How the thalidomide tragedy happened

The drug was introduced both as a sedative and also to help morning sickness of early pregnancy, which it undoubtedly did. As morning sickness is one of the first symptoms of pregnancy occurring in the first few weeks, the drug was obviously taken at the time potentially most disruptive to the developing fetus.

Due to strict control of drug marketing in the United States, the drug was never on sale there. However, it was still possible to obtain it there so cases of abnormal pregnancies due to thalidomide were encountered there.

Thalidomide quickly became widely used in many countries throughout the western world. It was in West Germany that a number of abnormal babies with certain characteristics were first recognized. The typical appearances were of absence or gross abnormalities of a limb or limbs, together with a red spot, similar to a Hindu caste-mark, between the eyebrows. Other abnormalities were subsequently identified including those of the bowel and kidneys and ear deformities. But these children were of normal intelligence.

At this time, nobody had made any connection between these abnormal babies and maternal ingestion of thalidomide during pregnancy. Thalidomide was available over the counter in West Germany; no prescription was required as it was thought to be so innocuous. A Dr Wilhelm Lenz sent out questionnaires to all the mothers of babies with these abnormalities enquiring about diet, health and drugs taken during pregnancy. Very few mentioned they had taken thalidomide, but when he reviewed the group asking specifically if they had taken it, virtually all answered in the

## Drugs and irradiation

affirmative; many obviously thought the drug so trivial it was not worth mentioning on the first occasion.

Further alarm bells sounded in Australia when an obstetrician who had been prescribing thalidomide to his patients noted the occurrence of these abnormal babies. Having established the link, the drug was quickly withdrawn. But during those few years, in the United Kingdom alone some 15 million thalidomide tablets were prescribed resulting in the birth of 329 abnormal children, many of whom have subsequently died.

In terms of pre-conceptual care, therefore, it is important to avoid taking medicines of any kind, wherever possible, and if consulting one's doctor, to advise him/her of the possibility of pregnancy. Inevitably mistakes occur, and drugs are taken during the early weeks of pregnancy often for very valid reasons. However, there are in fact very few drugs that we know to be definitely harmful to the developing fetus.

It is probably worthwhile to consider those drugs or groups of drugs that we know cause harm, and those that may be taken inadvertently or prescribed that are most likely to cause harm.

### CYTOTOXIC DRUGS

This group of drugs is definitely associated with causing abnormalities of the fetus. They are only used, however, in the treatment of leukaemia or other forms of cancer and never for pregnant women. Indeed, in the rare instance when a malignant condition is diagnosed during pregnancy, then the question of its termination must be considered if cytotoxic drugs are to be employed.

### ANTICONVULSANTS

These drugs are used in the treatment of epilepsy to prevent fits. It seems that there is a slightly higher malformation rate amongst babies born to mothers taking these preparations,

## Drugs and irradiation

but obviously the benefit of controlling epileptic fits is of much greater importance than the small risk of fetal abnormalities arising.

### ANTIBIOTICS

These are not uncommonly prescribed in pregnancy for urinary tract or chest infections. Although most are regarded as safe a few are to be avoided.

The tetracyclines have an ability to combine with calcium, and by crossing the placenta and combining into the developing fetal bones they can temporarily depress skeletal growth. No permanent damage is caused, however, as bone growth returns to normal once the drug is discontinued. Tetracyclines are better known for their ability to cause discoloration of infants' teeth. Depending on the stage of pregnancy at which the drug is taken, either the deciduous (baby) teeth or the permanent teeth may be affected. The yellow discoloration fades to brown and is permanent. In addition, the enamel of the teeth is poorly formed and there is a predisposition to dental caries.

Some of the antibiotics which have been used in the treatment of tuberculosis, in particular streptomycin, can cause hearing impairment or even deafness in the newborn, due to damage to the nerves responsible.

### ANALGESICS

Painkillers such as aspirin or paracetamol do not appear to be associated with any adverse effects on the fetus when taken in early pregnancy.

### ANTICOAGULANTS

These drugs are used to thin the blood either as a preventive or therapeutic measure in people who are at risk of, or have developed, blood clots in the veins – usually in the lower limbs. One of these drugs, warfarin, is known to cause abnormal development of the brain and face of the fetus in

## Drugs and irradiation

up to 30 per cent of cases when taken before the 12th week of pregnancy and should therefore be avoided.

The possibility of pregnancy should always be borne in mind when taking medication, and where doubt exists one's doctor should be aware of this so that if treatment is required the tried and trusted forms can be used.

Remember, virtually *all drugs* cross the placenta and enter the fetal circulation. Once this has happened then the ultimate effect on the fetus depends on many factors – the timing of the drug-taking in terms of the stage of pregnancy, the susceptibility of the fetus to damage, and the nature of the drug itself.

As illustrated with thalidomide, an important point is that the *fetus* may be affected by drugs that are *harmless to the mother*.

### Drug abuse and drug addiction

Drug abuse in pregnancy can be defined as the maternal administration of any chemical compound that causes adverse side-effects on mother and/or fetus. The definition, therefore, encompasses not only addictive drugs such as heroin, but any drug taken which has no obvious benefits in terms of treatment. I have already mentioned the commoner groups of drugs that may be taken during pregnancy, inadvertently in early pregnancy, and most of these offer little risk to the fetus. But what are the risks involved in maternal drug addiction?

#### HEROIN

Heroin is one of the most commonly abused narcotic drugs and its quality, price and purity vary. The drug carries a strong physical and psychological dependence, and the fetus will become as physically dependent as the mother.

The risks to the mother are well recognized, particularly in overdose, which may be fatal. Drug withdrawal is seldom fatal to the mother, but may result in miscarriage or death of the

## Drugs and irradiation

fetus. There is evidence to suggest that chromosomal abnormalities are commonest among the offspring of heroin addicts and certainly many types of congenital abnormality are found in these infants. However, associated environmental factors cannot be dissociated from heroin addiction as the underlying cause, making a simple cause and effect relationship difficult to establish.

MARIJUANA

The main maternal effect of this drug is euphoria and disorientation. One report from the United States suggested that it was used by 13 per cent of pregnant women. Marijuana use, together with alcohol abuse, is known to affect fetal growth and development and the use of both agents results in a large increase in the incidence of the fetal alcohol syndrome (see Chapter 5).

It is regarded as a soft drug, with less dependence and fewer side-effects, but its use should be avoided for the above reasons as well as for the possible conversion on to hard drugs.

LSD AND COCAINE

These drugs have similarly been reported as being associated with increased rates of congenital abnormality, although once again the issue is often clouded by associated factors.

## X-rays

Inadvertent exposure to X-irradiation during early pregnancy is not an uncommon situation and often leads to consultation and speculation regarding any harmful effect to the fetus. Indeed, termination of pregnancy may be sought on these grounds.

Much of the research on the effects of radiation on mother and fetus has arisen from studying the survivors of the atomic explosions at Hiroshima and Nagasaki in Japan at the end of

## Drugs and irradiation

the Second World War. These can hardly be compared with the small doses of radiation involved in diagnostic X-rays of the chest or abdomen. Obviously, the first 2 months of pregnancy are when the fetus is most susceptible to damage and while there exists a potential for causing adverse fetal effects, this has never been clearly shown with low-dose irradiation.

However, it is preferable to avoid unnecessary irradiation, so always consider the possibility of pregnancy prior to having an X-ray. During pregnancy, ultrasound has largely replaced X-rays as a diagnostic tool, but situations can arise where X-rays are indicated and these should not be excluded if the well-being of the mother is at stake.

The effects of multiple exposure to X-rays, as occurs in certain investigations of the kidneys or bowel, leads to increased concern regarding potential fetal damage, particularly when performed in early pregnancy. Even under these circumstances, however, it seems likely that if any gross fetal harm has been caused then the pregnancy will most probably result in a miscarriage, and that its continuation is an encouraging sign that no serious harm has been done.

# 7

# Infections and pregnancy

A certain proportion of abnormalities found in newborn babies is caused by infection during pregnancy. Many organisms are known to be implicated, so is there anything one can do to avoid them? In many cases, the answer is 'no', but in the instance of German measles or rubella infection, the answer is most certainly 'yes'.

During the summer of 1940 there was an epidemic of rubella infection throughout many parts of Australia. During the following spring a marked increase in the numbers of malformed babies born was noted, malformations principally involving the heart and eyes. By a retrospective analysis of these babies, a clear correlation was shown between congenital abnormality and rubella infection in early pregnancy. This was the first occasion on which it was appreciated that environmental, as well as genetic, factors could also be implicated in causing fetal abnormality.

**Rubella**

Rubella is a virus infection, and during the incubation period the virus circulates in the mother's bloodstream. It is readily able to cross the placenta and multiply in the fetal tissues. Once there, its main effect is to interfere in the process of cell division and disrupt the formation of the various organ systems. The determining factor as to whether it will cause fetal abnormality, and if so which type, is the stage of pregnancy at which the infection occurs. The earlier in

## Infections and pregnancy

pregnancy the infection takes place, the greater the likelihood of malformation.

When the infection occurs within the first 2 weeks following conception, the most likely outcome is that a miscarriage ensues and the embryo dies. Between the 4th and 6th weeks of pregnancy, infection is most likely to cause eye abnormalities, such as congenital cataract. From the 5th to 9th weeks, congenital heart defects are likely to be caused, and between the 8th and 12th, damage to the hearing mechanism is likely, resulting in congenital deafness (Table 7.1). The importance of the stage of pregnancy at which the infection occurs and what abnormalities are caused explains why deafness and blindness are seldom found together in the absence of heart disease, and that apart from deafness, isolated abnormalities are uncommon when the embryo has been infected prior to the 10th week of gestation.

**Table 7.1** Risk to fetus from rubella infection in pregnancy

| Gestation (weeks) | Effect | Incidence(%) |
|---|---|---|
| 2–4 | Miscarriage | 70–90 |
| 4–6 | Blindness | 30–70 |
| 5–9 | Congenital heart disease | 20–40 |
| 8–12 | Deafness | 10–25 |

Following further epidemics of rubella infection, it was demonstrated that the virus could still cause problems after the period of organ development was complete. Many other defects were found at birth including inflammation of the brain, heart and liver, together with mental retardation.

So what is the risk of having an abnormal baby following rubella infection during pregnancy? This has obviously been the cause of much investigation over the years, but results have varied widely. This may be due to variations in the

## Infections and pregnancy

virulence of the virus concerned, accuracy in diagnosing the condition or, in the case of deafness, follow-up of the affected children not continuing over a long enough period. Deafness, even in this day and age, may not be suspected during infancy. It is therefore possible only to give a rough idea as to the incidence of abnormalities occurring. Infection during the first few weeks of pregnancy presents a risk of between 30 and 70 per cent, during the second 4 weeks 25–55 per cent, during the third 4 weeks, 20–40 per cent, and during the fourth 4 weeks 10–25 per cent. The lower figure in each case is probably nearer to the true incidence.

Another study illustrated the problem from a slightly different angle, showing that when rubella infection occurred during the first three months of pregnancy congenital heart disease is 14 times as common, cataract 78 times as common, and deafness 40 times as common among their offspring as those born after a normal pregnancy. To put this in perspective, however, only about 2 per cent of congenital heart defects are attributable to rubella, and in less than 5 per cent of all abnormalities can rubella infection be implicated.

### PREVENTION

The reason for discussing this condition at such length is that it should be possible to prevent these serious fetal abnormalities from occurring at all, by ensuring one's immunity to rubella prior to pregnancy. Immunization may be acquired by exposure to the disease, and it is desirable for girls to have this exposure in childhood to confer immunity for the reproductive years of life.

Alternatively, vaccinations can be performed. The virus was first isolated in 1962 and by the early 1970s, a vaccine had been developed. It is effective and provides immunity for at least 4 years. At present, in this country vaccination is offered to girls at the age of 13 or 14, the rationale being to

## Infections and pregnancy

provide protection before the onset of the childbearing years. Routine vaccination of older women is not advocated because of the risk of pregnancy at the time of vaccination. However, older women who are potentially at risk of infection, such as teachers, nurses and midwives, may be vaccinated if found to be susceptible, with the advice not to become pregnant for 3 months following immunization.

Pregnant women are routinely tested for immunity to rubella in early pregnancy. The suggestion of active infection is grounds for termination of pregnancy under the Abortion Act of 1967. Pregnant women shown to be susceptible to rubella should be vaccinated following delivery.

The message is clear – ensure one's immunity to rubella *before* contemplating pregnancy. Many infections occurring during pregnancy can be harmful to the fetus, and unfortunately there is often little one can do to avoid them. But rubella *is* preventable.

### Other infections

A number of other infections, if contracted during pregnancy, can harm the fetus, but as I have said, in most instances there is little one can do to avoid them.

#### HERPES

The herpes simplex virus is the cause of cold sores but one particular type is commonly found in the female genital tract. Infections occurring in early pregnancy can result in miscarriage but one's main concern is infection of the fetus as it passes through the birth canal during labour. This can lead to severe infection of the newborn which may prove fatal, and under these circumstances the baby is often delivered by elective caesarean section.

It is important, therefore, that if there is a history of herpes infection, regular swabs are taken from the cervix and treatment commenced if necessary.

*Infections and pregnancy*

### TOXOPLASMOSIS AND CYTOMEGALOVIRUS (CMV)

Toxoplasmosis and cytomegalovirus are two other causes of congenital abnormality resulting from infection during pregnancy. They are relatively uncommon factors, so will not be discussed further here.

### AIDS

With the current publicity surrounding the increasing incidence of AIDS, it would be an omission not to give mention to this topic.

AIDS (acquired immune deficiency syndrome) is now known to result from infection with a virus (HIV). Certain groups of the population are known to be at greater risk of contracting the disease and these include male homosexuals or bisexuals, drug addicts and recipients of infected blood or blood products, such as haemophiliacs. It is now possible to detect the presence of an antibody to the AIDS virus, and although there might be some debate as to the wisdom of widespread screening of the population for this, the case for antibody testing is particularly strong in female drug addicts, female partners of drug addicts, or infected haemophiliacs or bisexual man. Such women should know they are not infected before becoming pregnant. Not only are HIV-antibody-positive women more likely to develop AIDS itself if they become pregnant, but there is also a high chance of the baby being infected and subsequently dying of AIDS.

# 8

# Medical history

Until now, we have considered some of the steps a healthy couple may wish to take prior to starting a pregnancy. Some women will be less fortunate by suffering from a condition that means pregnancy carries additional risks. Diabetes, thyroid gland disorders, heart and kidney disease, for example, can certainly be complicating factors where pregnancy is concerned, but today they are rarely contraindications.

## Diabetes

The diabetic, who requires insulin, is a good example of how the situation has improved. Prior to the introduction of insulin, some 60 years ago, a diabetic woman would have had little chance of becoming pregnant and if she did, then the chances of her surviving the pregnancy, let alone her baby surviving, were slim. Today, however, we can be much more optimistic. Pregnancy does result in increased doses of insulin being required, but by frequent checking of the blood glucose levels they can be maintained within the normal range. The better the control of the diabetes, then the better the chance of a successful outcome to the pregnancy.

One of the hazards of the diabetic pregnancy has been the increased incidence of abnormal babies born to these mothers. It now seems that this risk can be minimized by strict attention to control of the blood sugar levels in

*Medical history*

the pre-conceptual period and during the early weeks of pregnancy.

It is therefore imperative that diabetics are made aware of the implications of their condition with regard to pregnancy, and that control of their blood sugar levels is intensified for several months prior to conception in order to maximize the chances of a successful outcome. Most maternity hospitals have special clinics to supervise their diabetic mothers, where obstetrician and diabetic specialist can liaise and help maintain good control of the condition throughout pregnancy.

**Thyroid disorders**

Severe overactivity of the thyroid gland is often associated with lack of periods and infertility. So pregnancy is unlikely to occur before the condition is diagnosed, and if it does then it will probably result in miscarriage or premature delivery. Where drugs are being used to control the disease care must be taken that the dosage is not excessive, as these substances cross the placenta and can cause underactivity of the thyroid gland in the fetus, leading to impaired development of the fetus and mental retardation.

A deficiency of thyroxine, the hormone produced by the thyroid gland, is relatively uncommon in women of childbearing age, usually occurring in later life. However, when it does occur, there is often menstrual irregularity and impaired fertility. For those already on treatment for an underactive thyroid gland, it is important that the blood level of thyroxine is checked regularly, especially during pregnancy when the body's requirements for this hormone increase.

**Kidney disease**

There are, of course, many forms of kidney disease, of varying severity, which may or may not be associated with high blood

## Medical history

pressure. Today, except in the most severe cases, pregnancy is seldom considered dangerous, although the sufferer would still be well advised to seek a medical opinion prior to conception. It is worth bearing in mind that a condition which causes no symptoms under normal circumstances may worsen under the additional burden placed on the kidneys by pregnancy.

Patients undergoing treatment for their kidney disease such as dialysis (the artificial kidney) are able to conceive and should use contraceptives if they wish to avoid a pregnancy. There is, however, very little information available regarding this situation in terms of pregnancy outcomes.

Kidney transplants are becoming relatively common and any previous impairment of fertility is quickly restored following a successful operation. Adequate counselling is therefore necessary regarding the wisdom of pregnancy, and most authorities suggest an interval of 2 to 3 years following transplantation as safe. Certainly, pregnancy does not seem to cause any deterioration in kidney function under these circumstances.

**Heart disease**

Heart disease among women of the reproductive age group has become uncommon, mainly due to the dramatic reduction in the number of cases and the severity of rheumatic heart disease, the damage resulting from rheumatic fever. The use of antibiotics in the treatment of rheumatic fever has led to far fewer cases of rheumatic heart disease being seen, compared to 30 years ago.

Whatever the medical condition, therefore, it is most important to ascertain the implications with regard to pregnancy before conception. As I have stated, few illnesses are absolute contraindications to pregnancy but it is only sensible that medical advice is sought in good time.

# 9

# Infertility

So far we have considered aspects of general health that may require attention during the months prior to embarking on a pregnancy, assuming that conception will occur when anticipated. Unfortunately, in around 10 per cent of couples, this is not the case. Most healthy couples will have achieved a pregnancy within 12 to 18 months, and one would not normally consider undertaking investigations prior to this period of time. However, with increasing age, fertility does deteriorate and anxiety rises, in which case it may be appropriate to institute an examination and simple investigations earlier for reassurance.

**Causes of infertility**

Causes of failure to conceive can usually be attributed to four main categories (Table 9.1). In the case of the male partner, the reduction in number or complete absence of sperm is usually responsible and may be associated with reduced motility of those sperm present. Defective sperm production will therefore account for around 40 per cent of instances of impaired fertility.

The majority of the remainder of cases are due to some abnormality in the female reproductive system, either failure to produce an egg, damage to the Fallopian tubes, or some abnormality of the mucus produced by the neck of the womb which makes it hostile to sperm, killing them and preventing conception from occurring.

## Infertility

**Table 9.1** Causes of infertility

|  | % |
| --- | --- |
| Male factors | 30–40 |
| Erratic or absent egg production | 20 |
| Tubal damage or blockage | 20–30 |
| Cervical factors | 10 |
| Unexplained | 10 |

There may, of course, be elements of impaired fertility present in both partners, and indeed in around 10 per cent of couples no explanation can be found for their failure to conceive.

### Investigations

Most people will tend to be apprehensive regarding attending hospitals, particularly when the problem is as sensitive as failure to conceive. When the referral to a consultant is made, usually a gynaecologist, both partners should be encouraged to attend, not only to allay one another's anxieties but also to enable the doctor to take a history, examine both and explain to them the investigations and treatments available.

Usually, the initial consultation will involve no more than providing the doctor with details of the problem, and he will also want to know of any previous medical disorders. A general examination is usually carried out including a vaginal examination. Having spoken to and examined both partners, it is often then possible to hazard a guess at the likely underlying cause and institute the appropriate investigations, the commonest of which are described in Table 9.2.

# Infertility

**Table 9.2** Investigations of infertility

| Male | Female |
| --- | --- |
| History | History |
| Examination | Examination |
| Semen analysis | Temperature charts |
| | Blood tests |
| | Postcoital test |
| | Laparoscopy |
| | Hysterosalpingogram (see p. 65) |

## SEMEN ANALYSIS

This is the mainstay of investigation of the male partner, and he will normally be asked to submit two or three semen samples at monthly intervals to verify results. The normal values were mentioned in Chapter 2, but as a reminder the lower limits of normal are listed:

| | |
| --- | --- |
| Volume | 2 ml |
| Count | 20 million per ml |
| Motility | 50 per cent |
| Normal forms | more than 60 per cent |

## TEMPERATURE CHARTS

Temperature charts are designed to show whether or not a woman is ovulating. They rely on the principle that, following ovulation, there is an increased level of the hormone progesterone in the bloodstream, which produces a sustained rise in temperature during the second half of the menstrual cycle. The woman takes her temperature each morning before rising and plots it on a graph (Figure 9.1). These charts can be helpful in detecting ovulation and may also be useful if the couple wish to time sexual intercourse around this time of ovulation.

*Infertility*

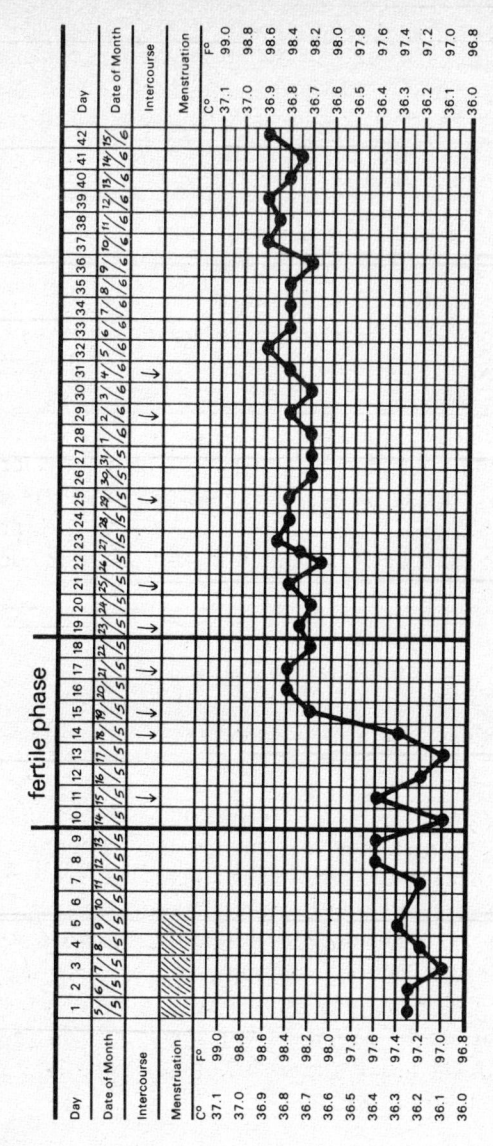

Fig. 9.1 Temperature chart demonstrating ovulation

## Infertility

Checking one's temperature each morning can become a chore, however, and particularly if the pattern is not obvious, as often happens, it is also depressing. It is much quicker to measure the actual progesterone level in the bloodstream at the appropriate time of the menstrual cycle.

BLOOD TESTS

A variety of investigations can be performed, some of which specifically assess the hormone status of the woman while others are designed to exclude the commoner general medical disorders.

*Full blood count*

This term describes the blood test which looks at the red and white blood cells and enables the doctor to diagnose anaemia or underlying infections.

*Thyroid gland function*

A variety of tests can assess how the thyroid gland is working, as either over activity or underactivity can be associated with impaired fertility.

*Rubella status*

It is important to know whether a woman has immunity to German measles before embarking on treatment designed to achieve a pregnancy. If no evidence of previous infection is detected, then immunization should be undertaken.

*Prolactin*

This is one of the hormones produced by the pituitary gland, situated at the base of the brain, and principally involved in the production of milk during breastfeeding when the level is grossly elevated. However, this situation can arise at other times for various reasons, and may reduce the chances of a pregnancy occurring.

*Progesterone*

As already mentioned, a high level of this hormone is indicative of ovulation having occurred.

*Infertility*

## Oestrogen

This is the other hormone produced by the ovary. There are several forms of oestrogen and it is sometimes useful to measure these as an assessment of how well the ovaries are working.

## FSH and LH

These two hormones, follicle stimulating hormone and luteinizing hormone, were mentioned in Chapter 2. Both are produced in the pituitary gland and control the function of the ovary including regulating egg production.

This is by no means an exhaustive list of blood tests available, and indeed some may not be performed at all. However, a great deal of information can be gathered from them.

### POSTCOITAL TEST

This test involves a sample of mucus from the neck of the womb being examined under a microscope, several hours following sexual intercourse. If few or no sperm are seen, or all appear dead, this may implicate cervical mucus as a causative factor in the couple's failure to conceive.

### LAPAROSCOPY

So far the investigations described are all relatively simple and straightforward. In many cases, however, the time arrives when it is necessary to inspect the uterus, ovaries and tubes to exclude any pelvic disease. Nowadays, the simplest way to do this is by a procedure called laparoscopy.

Laparoscopy is a minor operation performed under general anaesthetic where a telescope-like instrument is inserted into the abdominal cavity through a small cut just below the umbilicus. An excellent view of the pelvic organs can be obtained and any abnormality identified. The procedure may be performed on an outpatient basis but often involves an overnight stay in hospital.

*Infertility*

HYSTEROSALPINGOGRAM

This is dealt with more fully on p. 65.

## Treatments

DRUGS

So the investigations are completed. What treatment is available? Where the problem has been found to be faulty egg production drug treatments can be highly effective. The simplest of these comes in tablet form: clomiphene. It improves the chances of ovulation occurring at regular intervals with minimal risks of multiple pregnancy, by increasing the levels of FSH and LH.

Sometimes, however, it is necessary to boost the woman's own levels of FSH and LH by a course of these hormones by injections. This process must be very closely monitored to ensure that the ovaries are not overstimulated and result in multiple pregnancy.

TUBAL SURGERY

In the case of tubal damage then tubal surgery may be considered. This involves a major operation to try and restore the tubes to normal. But even with the most skilled surgeon, 100 per cent success cannot be guaranteed.

*IN VITRO* FERTILIZATION (IVF)

Where tubal surgery proves unsuccessful, or where the extent of tubal disease is too extensive to contemplate any surgical correction, then today the question of *in vitro* fertilization (test tube baby) may be considered. This is a complicated and expensive form of treatment and at best offers only a 10–15 per cent chance of success. It is to be hoped that over the coming years, however, this will be improved upon and enable the technique to offer higher pregnancy rates.

*Infertility*

### ARTIFICIAL INSEMINATION BY DONOR (AID)

The use of certain drugs to alter the quality of the cervical mucus may sometimes be employed, but it is in this area and that of a poor sperm count that treatment is most difficult. Many measures have been tried to improve the sperm count but none have met with any significant degree of success. Under these circumstances, the couple may feel they wish to attempt artificial insemination by donor (AID) but this is charged with many problems, both technical and psychological.

### GIFT

One recent development in the treatment of infertility has been the technique known as GIFT – or gamete intrafallopian transfer. Here, the eggs and sperm are placed together in the Fallopian tube and fertilization allowed to occur naturally. However, the woman must have healthy tubes to enable the procedure to be performed, and although it is in its early days of development this technique holds some promise.

As mentioned at the start of this chapter, in around 10 per cent of couples no cause can be found for their failure to conceive. In others, treatment has failed. Then there arises the most difficult decision for both the couple and their doctor, that of when to pursue the problem no further.

# 10

# Genetic considerations

As already stated, around 2 per cent of all babies are born with a serious abnormality of one kind or another. Once the initial shock and distress of such an occurrence has subsided, the parents will invariably wonder what caused the abnormality and what the chances are of any further children they might have being similarly affected.

Perhaps it would be worthwhile first outlining a few principles regarding human genetics before considering the question of genetic counselling and the various techniques of prenatal diagnosis – detecting abnormalities of the fetus in early pregnancy.

## Chromosomes

Every cell in the human body contains its complement of chromosomes. These are the structures that carry the genetic information responsible for an individual's appearance and characteristics. All living organisms have their own specific number of chromosomes per cell and a few of these are shown in Table 10.1. In humans, the normal chromosome complement is 46, occurring as 23 pairs of chromosomes. The exception to this number of chromosomes is in the sperm and ovum, these having only 23 chromosomes each. Thus, when fertilization occurs and the sperm fuses with the ovum, the correct chromosome number is arrived at. The first 22 pairs of chromosomes are called 'autosomes' while the last pair are responsible for the sex of the person and

## Genetic considerations

known as the 'sex chromosomes'. When seen through the microscope, chromosomes can be accurately put into their appropriate pairs; because of their appearance, the sex chromosomes are called X or Y. In a female, a cell is composed of 44 autosomes and two X chromosomes, while in the male a cell consists of 44 autosomes plus one X and one Y chromosome. Figure 10.1 shows how the sex of a baby is determined.

**Table 10.1** Chromosome distribution

| Cucumber | 14 | Rabbit | 44 |
|---|---|---|---|
| Tomato | 24 | Man | 46 |
| Bee | 32 | Horse | 66 |
| Snail | 54 | Pigeon | 80 |

GENES

Genes are distributed along the length of the chromosomes and are composed of a substance called DNA (deoxyribonucleic acid). Genes, like chromosomes, exist in pairs, one of each pair being contributed by each parent. It is through this mixing of the genes that parental characteristics may be expressed in their children. There are thousands of genes and only 23 pairs of chromosomes, so obviously each chromosome carries thousands of genes.

## Genetic abnormalities

As said before, every couple worries that their baby might be abnormal. It is worth bearing in mind, though, that none of us is perfect and we all have minor abnormalities of one kind or another such as short legs or big ears. Congenital abnormalities occur over a wide range of degrees of severity and we can classify these as minimal, moderate and severe.

## Genetic considerations

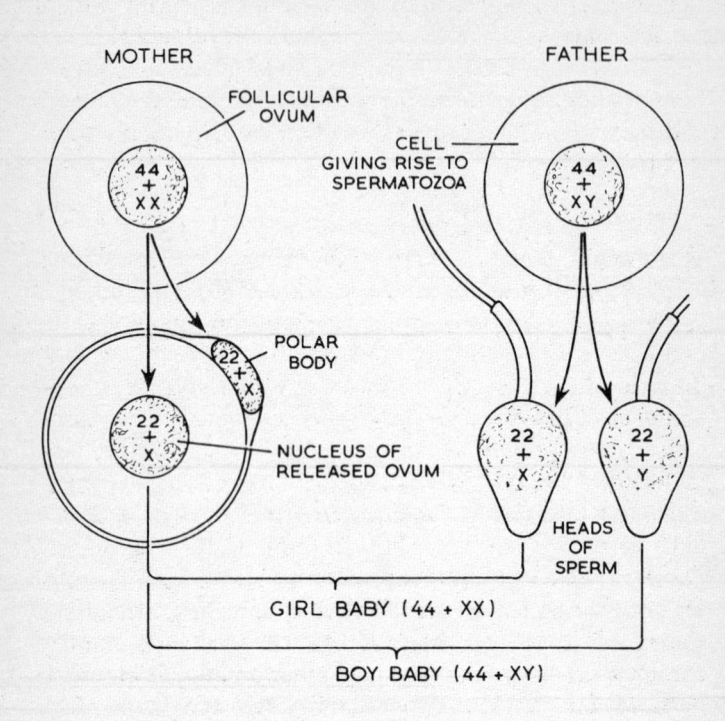

Fig. 10.1 How a baby's sex is determined

Minimal abnormalities include extra or fused fingers and toes, or birthmarks, which may require only minor surgical treatment. This sort of defect arises approximately 1 in every 100 babies.

Moderate abnormalities, such as cleft palate and hare lip, congenital dislocation of the hip and some forms of congenital heart disease are usually readily dealt with by surgery. Following this, a completely normal life can be anticipated

## Genetic considerations

for the child. This group also has a similar incidence affecting 1 in 100 infants.

The severe abnormalities are incompatible with normal life and may result in the early death of the infant. They are not normally amenable to surgery and include such conditions as Down's syndrome, congenital absence of the kidneys and severe heart abnormalities. These, too, generally occur in 1 in 100 babies.

INTRINSIC ABNORMALITIES

When considering the causes of these abnormalities, we can divide them into extrinsic (environmental) and intrinsic (congenital). We have already discussed many of the extrinsic factors earlier in this book – smoking, alcohol, drugs and nutrition. In this chapter we are concerned with the intrinsic group – congenital inherited factors. The reason why certain abnormalities are inherited is not clearly understood, but the study of genetics advances each year and ultimately may clarify the situation.

### Down's syndrome

One of the commonest genetic disorders is Down's syndrome (mongolism). In these cases, each cell contains an extra chromosome, 47 instead of 46, and the condition is known to be more common with increasing maternal age (Table 10.2). Other chromosomal disorders also increase with age, and in the late thirties the likelihood of any chromosomal abnormality occurring is in the order of 1 in 70. As shown in Table 10.2, where genetic abnormalities are known to have previously occurred the risks are increased. Genetic counsellors can advise of the risks of such conditions occurring or recurring, and any prospective parents who worry that they may have a problem should seek pre-pregnancy advice from a genetic clinic. In the vast majority of cases, their suspicions will be allayed.

*Genetic considerations*

**Table 10.2**  Risk of Down's syndrome related to age of mother

| Maternal age | No previously affected child | One previously affected child |
|---|---|---|
| under 25 | less than 1 in 1000 | 1 in 200 |
| 26–30 | 1 in 800 | 1 in 200 |
| 31–35 | 1 in 500 | 1 in 200 |
| 37 | 1 in 250 | 1 in 125 |
| 39 | 1 in 150 | 1 in 75 |
| 40 | 1 in 100 | 1 in 50 |
| 41 | 1 in 80 | 1 in 40 |
| 42 | 1 in 60 | 1 in 30 |
| 43 | 1 in 50 | 1 in 25 |
| 44 | 1 in 40 | 1 in 20 |

**Prenatal diagnosis**

While it is useful for prospective parents to be aware of the risks of abnormalities occurring, they will also want to know, having embarked on a pregnancy, if their unborn child is normal. Great advances have been made in this field of prenatal diagnosis, detecting abnormalities before birth and these are considered next.

ULTRASOUND SCANS

The technique of using high frequency sound waves is now virtually routine in every maternity hospital and comprises part of normal antenatal care. The technology of these machines has become increasingly sophisticated so that very precise images of the fetus can be obtained and its anatomy more closely examined.

Most hospitals perform an ultrasound scan on all mothers, often at around 16 to 18 weeks of pregnancy. At this stage, it

## Genetic considerations

should be possible to examine closely the baby's brain, spine, heart, kidneys, bladder and intestines, as well as limbs.

### AMNIOCENTESIS

Ultrasound, of course, cannot identify genetic abnormalities unless there is an obvious physical defect present. To assess the chromosome make-up of the fetus we must obtain cells from it, and this can be achieved by a procedure known as amniocentesis. This entails withdrawing a small volume of amniotic fluid, the fluid which surrounds the baby within the womb, and obtaining the cells in this which are fetal in origin. By examining these one can identify any chromosomal abnormality as well as determining the sex of the baby.

The procedure is performed under ultrasound guidance at around 16 weeks gestation, but is not without risk as there is a small chance (1 in 150) that it may precipitate a miscarriage. It is performed, therefore, usually only where there is a good indication such as increasing maternal age, previously affected babies, or a family history of abnormalities.

### CHORIONIC VILLUS SAMPLING

The problem with amniocentesis is that it cannot be performed until the 16th week of pregnancy. As the results of the chromosome analysis may take 3 or 4 weeks to obtain, if a serious abnormality if found to exist and a termination of pregnancy is necessary, the procedure carries far greater risks. A relatively new technique called chorionic villus sampling can be performed between 8 and 12 weeks of pregnancy and involves taking a small sample of the fetal cells from the developing placenta. Once again, the chromosomal complement of the fetus can be examined and the pregnancy terminated at an earlier stage if there appears to be a lethal abnormality.

### FETOSCOPY

This, too, is a relatively new technique, whereby a small

## *Genetic considerations*

telescope-like instrument is passed into the womb and the fetus is directly visualized. Abnormalities can be identified and a sample of blood can be taken from the fetus for analysis. This procedure, however, is not widely available and does carry substantial risk of miscarriage or premature delivery.

### The results

Firstly, no couple should feel pressurized into having these investigations. They should be told what is involved and associated risks. Most importantly, the couple should consider their attitude to termination of pregnancy if an abnormality is demonstrated. This is, of course, both a highly charged issue and a moral dilemma. Adequate counselling and support is essential should an abnormality be found; there will be many factors influencing the couple, and no easy solution for them.

# 11

# Previous obstetric experience

Happily, most women progress through pregnancy uneventfully. Inevitably, however, unforeseen circumstances can arise which may cast doubt in the minds of a couple regarding the wisdom of contemplating a further pregnancy. It might be useful, therefore, to consider these situations and offer some form of reassurance where appropriate.

**Miscarriage**

Technically speaking, the medical profession refer to a miscarriage as a 'spontaneous abortion'. Abortion, however, is a word which, in the minds of many people, conjures up an aura of criminal interference or legal termination of pregnancy and is therefore little used outside medical practice. The dictionary definition of a spontaneous abortion is, 'expulsion of the fetus before the 28th week of pregnancy'; this is still the gestational age before which, legally, the fetus is not considered viable. It is not all that uncommon today for very small infants delivered at 26 or 27 weeks gestation to survive, thanks to the great advances in the skills and techniques employed in special care baby nurseries.

Miscarriages tend to be divided into two groups, early and late: early occurring before the 14th week of pregnancy; and late after this stage. Early miscarriages are probably much more common than we suspect. The frequency of recognized early miscarriage in the general population has been estimated to range between 15 and 20 per cent. The actual rate is difficult to determine, as in some cases women will miscarry completely at home and not need to seek medical help. Indeed, in many instances, a miscarriage may not even be recognized, and be mistaken for a delayed or heavier than normal period. Consequently, many experts feel the true rate of early miscarriage may be closer to 30–50 per cent of pregnancies.

CAUSES OF MISCARRIAGE

It is often difficult to identify the actual cause of a single miscarriage, but in general terms we know the possible causes and these are shown in Table 11.1. While early miscarriage is thought most commonly to be due to genetic or immunological factors, later miscarriages are more usually due to abnormalities of the womb or neck of the womb. Any serious infection during pregnancy can precipitate a miscarriage or premature delivery, as can chronic maternal illness.

**Table 11.1** Causes of miscarriage

Genetic factors
Immunological factors
Maternal disease
Infections
Uterine abnormalities
External factors

Exposure to radiation is known to induce miscarriage in animal studies, but its effects on human pregnancy are less well known. Certain drugs, cigarette smoking and alcohol abuse have all been implicated in early pregnancy loss; however, there is a wide variation in the ability of an early pregnancy to survive these abuses and it is most likely that many factors are involved.

## Previous obstetric experience

WHAT CAN BE DONE?

Miscarriage is a sufficiently common occurrence for there to be no cause for alarm. Inevitably such events cause distress, but one can be reassured by the fact that there is every likelihood of a subsequent pregnancy progressing entirely normally. For this reason, no specific investigations are necessary. If, however, a woman suffers repeated miscarriages, say three or more consecutive pregnancies, this is called 'recurrent abortion' and merits closer study.

Any investigations should commence with a full history being elicited from the woman, together with a physical (including vaginal) examination. Certain blood tests may throw some light on the problem, such as in the case of an underactive thyroid gland, when the thyroxine levels in the blood will be low. Another useful blood test is to look at the chromosomes of both partners to determine if there is any genetic abnormality that prevents them conceiving a viable pregnancy (see also Chapters 9 and 10). Tests to exclude any occult infection can be performed in case this is a contributory factor.

If an abnormality of the womb itself is suspected, then a hysterosalpingogram can be performed. This is a type of X-ray investigation where dye is injected through the neck of the womb to fill the cavity of the uterus and demonstrate any abnormality in shape or size. No anaesthetic is usually required and the test takes only a few minutes to perform. Thereafter, surgical treatment may be indicated.

In the absence of any demonstrable anatomical or chromosomal abnormality, attention is being focused increasingly on an immunological factor being to blame. In other words, the mother is unable to recognize the fetus as her own and rejects it, resulting in miscarriage, in much the same way as transplanted organs such as hearts or kidneys may be rejected. Further investigation into this area may result in some further treatment, but for the time being we must await developments.

## Tubal or ectopic pregnancy

Another cause of early pregnancy loss is ectopic pregnancy. In this situation, the embryo implants in a site outside the uterus, most commonly in the Fallopian tube. There is, of course, insufficient space for the embryo to develop and the pregnancy terminates, usually at around 6 to 10 weeks gestation, either by being expelled from the end of the Fallopian tube, and/or bursting the tube which may result in severe internal bleeding.

In the United Kingdom, tubal pregnancy is said to occur in 1 in 300 pregnancies so is not especially common. Factors which predispose to this happening are shown in Table 11.2.

**Table 11.2** Predisposing factors of tubal pregnancy

> Previous tubal damage
>   infection
>   surgery
>   sterilization
> Intrauterine contraceptive device (coil)
> Progesterone only pill (minipill)
> Previous tubal pregnancy

The treatment will often be surgical in order to arrest the bleeding, and may involve removal of the portion of the tube containing the pregnancy.

Statistically, there is an increased chance of a woman having another tubal pregnancy, although more often than not any subsequent pregnancy will be within the womb (intrauterine). The significance therefore, in terms of pre-

## Previous obstetric experience

conceptual advice, is that these women should be aware that in future pregnancies they consult a doctor in the early weeks to confirm that the pregnancy is in the right place.

**Previous infant loss**

Any parents who have suffered the grief of a previous stillborn infant or baby dying shortly following delivery will naturally be anxious regarding the outcome of future pregnancies. Advice is obviously based on the cause of the previous tragedy and these can be broadly divided into either fetal or maternal causes.

Obviously, if the baby was abnormal then one can usually offer prediction of the likelihood of recurrence, and tests in subsequent pregnancy to confirm the normality of the fetus. These are discussed in more detail in Chapter 10.

As mentioned in Chapter 1, prematurity is the other main factor in perinatal mortality. Premature labour and delivery may occur for many of the same reasons as miscarriage, such as infection or abnormalities of the uterus or cervix; or premature delivery may be deliberately undertaken if the health of mother and/or fetus is in question. Such situations arise, for example, if the mother's blood pressure rises to very high levels (pre-eclampsia), the placenta separates prematurely (placental abruption), or there is doubt as to how well the placenta is working in providing the fetus with adequate nutrition to allow growth (placental insufficiency).

Most of these circumstances, however, are unlikely to recur. The suspicion of the neck of the womb being weakened (cervical incompetence) may raise the question of a stitch being inserted to keep it closed, and this can either be done prior to pregnancy or more usually when the pregnancy has advanced to the 3 or 4 month stage.

Anyone who has previously lost a baby will be kept under close supervision during subsequent pregnancies. Monitoring

*Previous obstetric experience*

of the fetus and its growth using techniques such as ultrasound helps to provide reassurance and an ultimately successful outcome of pregnancy.

**Previous abnormal deliveries**

Obstetricians are increasingly being taken to task about intervention during labour, rather than allowing what is essentially a natural process to occur naturally. I would like to think that most obstetricians are happy to allow labour to occur naturally, but we must be alert to when labour becomes abnormal and take the necessary steps to correct the situation. Thus, forceps deliveries and caesarean sections occur, in the hope of securing a healthy mother and child at the end of the day.

Forceps deliveries are very common amongst first labours, and unusual subsequently. This is because the pelvic tissues have never been stretched before, and the quality of the uterine contractions are less good. Except under unusual circumstances, most mothers who have undergone a forceps delivery of their first child can be reassured that it will be completely normal the second time around.

Caesarean sections obviously carry more significance in terms of subsequent delivery. The uterus bears a scar, a potential weak spot which may burst during labour. In general terms, therefore, if the caesarean was performed for a non-recurring condition then there is a prospect of achieving a normal delivery subsequently; but if the indication for a caesarean is a recurrent problem – such as a small pelvis – further deliveries will probably be by caesarean section. Of course, it is impossible to generalize so these worries regarding future pregnancies should be discussed with one's family doctor or obstetrician.

# 12

# Sexual problems

Although this is difficult to quantify in terms of frequency, the medical profession is increasingly aware nowadays of difficulties arising in relation to sexual intercourse. It seems reasonable, therefore, to mention the commoner ones here and discuss briefly what can be done to help these situations.

## Problems affecting males

### POOR LIBIDO

A loss of interest in sex tends to be a less common complaint from men than women. A commoner male complaint is of problems with arousal or ejaculation, but reduced interest may be related to the particular partner involved or with physical or psychological disorders.

### IMPOTENCE

The inability to achieve or maintain an erection is one of the commonest male sexual problems. When due to a physical condition the onset may be gradual, whereas if psychological factors are involved it may be sudden.

### PREMATURE EJACULATION

This term is rather ill-defined as, apart from the case where ejaculation occurs prior to penetration, there is no specific time limit to the duration of intercourse prior to ejaculation. This condition is particularly common among young males, and is almost always attributable to psychological factors.

## Sexual problems

RETARDED EJACULATION

This is a problem of inability or difficulty in ejaculating and is not particularly common. It is said to be typical in inhibited men, and may only occur with a partner, or be so marked as to make ejaculation impossible even by masturbation.

PAIN ON EJACULATION

This is an uncommon problem which may be due to spasm of the perineal muscles.

## Problems affecting females

IMPAIRED LIBIDO

This is the commonest sexual problem among women. It may occur either as a result of longstanding inhibitions about sex, or of specific problems with general relationships.

IMPAIRED AROUSAL

This implies that a woman begins to get aroused but for some reason this causes anxiety which in turn prevents further arousal.

DIFFICULTIES IN ATTAINING ORGASM

This can be divided into cases where this has never been achieved, and those where it has occurred under other circumstances, such as masturbation, but not with a partner.

VAGINISMUS

This term describes the spasm of the pelvic muscles surrounding the vagina when penetration is attempted which renders intercourse impossible.

DYSPAREUNIA

This is the medical term applied to pain during intercourse. Depending on the site of the pain, it is defined as either superficial or deep. It can result from local causes such as poor lubrication, or scarring of the vagina from previous

## Sexual problems

childbirth, or may be caused by more generalized conditions affecting the pelvis.

## Causes

### PSYCHOLOGICAL FACTORS

These tend to arise either because of factors such as sexual inhibitions stemming from a sheltered upbringing, or as a result of some precipitating factor such as childbirth or physical illness. Subsequent anxiety and apprehension regarding sexual activity further compounds the problem.

### PHYSICAL FACTORS

Sexual difficulties arise not uncommonly in association with illness – either as a direct result of the condition itself, or as a consequence of the treatment prescribed, either surgical or medical in the form of drugs. A good example is diabetes. Studies have shown that 35–60 per cent of diabetic men have problems achieving an erection, and many also have ejaculatory problems. It has been suggested that women diabetics may have problems related to sexual responsiveness.

Many medications are known to interfere with sexual function, the commoner being some drugs used in the control of blood pressure, some types of tranquillizers, and even the oral contraceptive pill. The effects of alcohol on sexual performance are well recognized.

## Treatment

The majority of sexual problems can be helped merely through consulting one's general practitioner or gynaecologist. As with the problem of infertility, it is important that the matter be tackled through discussion with both partners. Reassurance, education and identification of any relevant factors will often be all that is necessary.

## Sexual problems

Obviously, more involved forms of sex therapy may sometimes be needed, *à la* Masters and Johnson, but this is best dealt with by referral to an experienced sex therapist.

As sexual problems are not uncommon, society should adopt the maxim of prevention being better than cure, and adequate sex education in adolescence may play an important role in this area.

# 13

# The early weeks

So far we have considered various areas to which attention can be focused with the intention of maximizing the chances of a successful pregnancy. In concluding this book, let us look at the course of the early weeks of pregnancy, the changes that will occur and mention some of the commoner problems.

### Amenorrhoea – absence of periods

In women who have regular periods the commonest cause for a missed period is pregnancy. This is usually the first sign to the woman that she has conceived – as we already know, even 10 to 14 days after a missed period fetal development is already well underway.

In cases where periods tend to be erratic or if menstruation has not recommenced following a previous delivery or while breastfeeding, the picture may be confused and the diagnosis of pregnancy not made for some time.

### Breast changes

Breast tenderness and fullness with tingling in the nipples are common early symptoms of pregnancy and usually occur within 5 or 6 weeks of the last menstrual period. The veins under the breast skin become more prominent, and the nipples become more pigmented and appear darker. These changes tend to be more marked in first pregnancies.

*The early weeks*

**Morning sickness**

Nausea and vomiting are well-known symptoms of pregnancy but are by no means universal. Probably 50–60 per cent of women experience some degree of morning sickness, which normally starts 5 or 6 weeks after the missed period. The situation usually improves after the first 3 months of pregnancy, but some people have persistent problems throughout it.

Occasionally, the sickness and vomiting can be so severe as to lead to dehydration and admission to hospital is required. This condition is known as hyperemesis gravidarum. Drugs to help prevent one being sick (antiemetics), are available but after the scare surrounding the drug Debendox possibly causing fetal abnormalities (not to mention thalidomide), these have become less widely used and are reserved for extreme situations.

**Other complaints**

Another annoyance in early pregnancy is often the necessity to frequently empty one's bladder – known as frequency in the medical profession. Constipation and tiredness are also common complaints. Frequency and constipation often persist throughout pregnancy, but the feeling of tiredness is often replaced by a feeling of well-being in later pregnancy.

**Confirmation of pregnancy**

The history of a missed period, together with the other symptoms of pregnancy, may make any other confirmatory test unnecessary. However, conclusive proof can be obtained from a urine test which depends on the presence of the hormone hCG (human chorionic gonadotrophin). This is the hormone produced by the developing placenta, the

## The early weeks

trophoblast. Remember, therefore, a positive test need not necessarily mean the presence of a viable pregnancy, merely the presence of a viable trophoblast.

Ultrasound scans are extremely helpful in confirming pregnancy and its viability. From about 6 or 7 weeks after the last period, the fetal heart may be seen beating, and the pregnancy can be dated where doubt exists by measuring the length of the fetus

**Common problems**

Pain arising in the lower abdomen, backache and vaginal bleeding are not uncommon occurrences in early pregnancy and need not necessarily reflect adversely on the outcome of the pregnancy.

Pain, of course, is a very subjective feature. As the uterus enlarges, some degree of discomfort is to be expected and need only be of concern if it progresses to a greater severity when medical advice should be sought.

We have mentioned the problem of miscarriages earlier and it is important to remember that bleeding in early pregnancy is termed as some form of abortion by the medical profession. Scanty bleeding, therefore, is termed a threatened abortion; this may resolve or progress to an inevitable abortion – a miscarriage. It is reassuring to know that a pregnancy continuing after bleeding in early pregnancy will invariably produce a healthy normal baby. Bleeding, however, cannot be regarded as normal and should be reported to one's doctor for further assessment.

# 14

# Conclusion

As the costs of running the National Health Service soar year by year, more and more emphasis has been placed on the role of preventive medicine. Pregnancy has for some years now been regarded as an ideal opportunity of promoting health care within what is an essentially captive population of women. The logical extension of this is to health care prior to pregnancy with the hope of improving the health of the population in general and further reducing the perinatal mortality rate. While these are worthy motives, it is extremely difficult to attribute their success to pre-pregnancy care alone. Any measures to improve one's health, however, seem common sense and are to be commended.

I have tried to outline those areas that I see as important for women preparing for pregnancy for the first time, and have tried to offer reassurance to those whose previous pregnancies have had an unsatisfactory outcome.

Preconceptual care is becoming increasingly recognized by the medical profession as an important area, and it is to be hoped that with this acceptance preconceptual advice clinics will become available to wider sectors of the general public.

# Glossary

**amenorrhoea**  Absence of periods

**amniocentesis**  The procedure whereby a fine needle is introduced through the abdominal wall into the womb, enabling one to withdraw a sample of the amniotic fluid that surrounds the fetus; by this technique, certain abnormalities of the fetus can be detected

**amniotic fluid**  The fluid within the pregnancy sac that surrounds the fetus

**autosomes**  The non-sex chromosomes of which there are 22 pairs

**blastocyst**  One stage of the developing embryo

**cataract**  The condition where the lens in the eye becomes opaque and leads to blindness

**chorionic villus sampling**  A technique performed in early pregnancy whereby small portions of the developing placenta can be obtained by passing a fine needle through the neck of the womb; this provides an alternative to amniocentesis in the diagnosis of fetal abnormality

**chromosomes**  the paired strands of DNA in the cell nucleus that carry the genetic code

**corpus luteum**  The site on the ovary from which ovulation has occurred

**decidua**  The thickened, developed endometrium

**ectopic pregnancy**  When the pregnancy implants at a site outside the womb, most commonly in the Fallopian tube

**endometrium**  The layer of cells which comprise the lining of the womb

## Glossary

**Fallopian tube** Also called oviduct, this is the structure along which the egg, released by the ovary, travels to the womb, and here fertilization occurs

**fetal alcohol syndrome** A group of abnormalities found in the offspring of mothers with a high alcohol intake

**FSH** (follicle stimulating hormone) One of the hormones produced by the pituitary gland, at the base of the brain, which stimulates the ovaries to develop follicles, one of which releases an egg each menstrual cycle

**follicle** The small cyst-like structure that arises on the surface of the ovary and contains the egg (ovum)

**hyperemesis gravidarum** Excessive sickness and vomiting in pregnancy

**hypothalamus** A part of the brain that controls the pituitary gland's secretion of hormones

**IUCD** The intrauterine contraceptive device or coil

**LH** (luteinizing hormone) The hormone produced by the pituitary gland, responsible for causing ovulation

**morula** A stage of development of the embryo, comprising a clump of cells, which proceeds to become the blastocyst

**neural tube defect** A collective term referring to developmental abnormalities of the fetal central nervous system; an example is spina bifida

**oestrogen** One of the female sex hormones produced by the ovary

**organogenesis** The term used to describe the process of development of the various organ systems within the growing embryo

**ovulation** The process whereby the mature follicle on the surface of the ovary ruptures, releasing an egg

**ovum** The egg

**perinatal mortality rate** An expression of the number of babies lost either as stillbirths or deaths in the first week of life

**pill** The oral contraceptive pill

*Glossary*

**pituitary gland**   A small gland at the base of the brain that secretes hormones responsible for the control of menstruation, ovulation and lactation

**placenta** (the afterbirth)   The structure that enables nutrients to be transferred from fetus to mother

**placental abruption**   Also called placentae abruptio, this is premature separation of the placenta from the wall of the womb

**placenta praevia**   Where the placenta has implanted in the lower part of the womb and can cause profuse vaginal bleeding

**pre-eclampsia**   Very high blood pressure in pregnancy

**progesterone**   One of the female sex hormones produced by the ovary

**prolactin**   A hormone produced by the pituitary gland, primarily responsible for control of lactation

**rubella**   German measles

**sex chromosomes**   Termed X and Y, XX representing a normal female, and XY a normal male

**spermatogenesis**   The process of sperm production

**spontaneous abortion**   Miscarriage

**therapeutic abortion**   Termination of pregnancy

**ultrasound**   The technique of visualizing the contents of the uterus by sound waves

**uterus**   The womb

# Index

abnormal deliveries, previous, 68
abortion, spontaneous, 63
AID (artificial insemination by donor), 55
AIDS, 44
alcohol, 30–2
  abuse, and pregnancy, 31–2
  effects on pregnancy, 31
  fetal syndrome, 31
  historical background, 30
  paternal drinking, 32
amenorrhoea, 17, 73
amniocentesis, 3, 61
analgesics, 36
antibiotics, 36
anticoagulants, 36
anticonvulsants, 35–6
arousal, impaired in females, 70
artificial insemination by donor (AID), 55
autosomes, 56

blood tests, for infertility, 52–3
  full count, 52
breast changes, 73–4

cadmium, mercury, lead, 24–5
Caesarean section, 68
carbohydrates, 20
chorionic villus sampling, 3, 61
chromosome, 56–7
  autosomes, 56
  distribution, 57
  fetal abnormalities, 3
cocaine, 38
conception, 9–11

contraception, 13–16
  combined pill, 13–14
  intrauterine contraceptive device (IUCD), 15–16
  progesterone-only pill, 15
corpus luteum, 8
cytomegalovirus (CMV), 44
cytotoxic drugs, 35

diabetes, 45–6
diet, 17–26
  carbohydrates, 20
  essential nutrients, 21
  fats, 20
  minerals and trace elements, 23–5
    cadmium, mercury, lead, 24–5; iodine, 24; iron, 23; zinc, 23–4
  proteins, 20
  supplementation, 25–6
  vitamins, 21–3
    A, 21–2; B complex, 22; C, D, 22
Down's syndrome, 59–60
  and mother's age, 60
drugs, 33–8
  abuse and addiction, 37–8
    heroin, 37–8
    LSD and cocaine, 38
    marijuana, 38
  adverse effects on fetus, 33–7
    analgesics, 36; antibiotics, 36; anticoagulants, 36; anticonvulsants, 35–6; cytotoxic, 35; thalidomide, 33–5

*81*

# Index

treatment for infertility, 54
Dutch Hunger Winter, 18
dyspareunia, 70–1

early weeks, in pregnancy, 73–5
  amenorrhoea, 73
  breast changes, 73–4
  confirmation of pregnancy, 74–5
  common problems, 75
  frequency, 74
  morning sickness, 74
ectopic (tubal) pregnancy, 66–7
ejaculation problems, 69–70
endometrium, 8
essential nutrients, 21

Fallopian tubes, 9, 10, 15
  pregnancy in, 66–7
fats, 20
fertilization, *in vitro*, 54
fetal abnormalities, 2–3
  chromosome, 3
fetal alcohol syndrome, 24, 30, 31
fetal development, 5–12
fetoscopy, 61–2
fetus,
  development, 11–12
    times, 10
  external characteristics, 11
follicle stimulating hormone (FSH), 5, 9
  test, 53
food deprivation, 17–18
forceps deliveries, 68

gamete intrafallopian transfer (GIFT), 55
genes, 57–9
  determining sex, 58
genetics, 56–62
  abnormalities, 57–9
  chromosomes, 56–7
  Down's syndrome, 59
  prenatal diagnosis, 60–2
    results of, 62
GIFT, 55

health, and smoking, 27–8
heart disease, 47
height and weight, ideal, 19
heroin, 37–8
herpes, 43
hormones,
  follicle stimulating (FSH), 5, 9, 53
  human chorionic gonadotrophin (hCG), 74
  luteinizing (LH), 5, 9, 53
hypothalamus, 5
hysterosalpingogram, 54

immunization, against rubella, 42
impotence, 69
infant loss, previous, 67–8
infections, and pregnancy, 40–4
  AIDS, 44
  cytomegalovirus (CMV), 44
  herpes, 43
  rubella, 40–3
    prevention, 42–3; risk to fetus, 41
  toxoplasmosis, 44
infertility, 48–55
  causes of, 48
  investigations for, 49–50
    blood tests, 52–3; semen analysis, 50; temperature charts, 50, 51; treatments, 54–5
intrauterine contraceptive device (IUCD), 15–16
*in vitro* fertilization, 54
iodine, 24
iron, 23
irradiation, 38–9
  X-rays, 38–9
    Hiroshima, Nagasaki, 38

kidney disease, 46–7

laparoscopy, 53
Leningrad, siege of, 17
libido, poor, 69, 70

# Index

living standards, improvements in, 1–2
LSD, 38
luteinizing hormone (LH), 5, 9
  test, 53

MAFF survey, 24
marijuana, 38
medical history, 45–7
  diabetes, 45–6
  heart disease, 46–7
  kidney disease, 46–7
  thyroid disorders, 46
men,
  and effects of smoking on, 29
  sexual problems affecting, 69–70
  paternal drinking, 32
menstrual cycle, 5–8
menstruation:
  control of, 6
  events leading to, 8
  and ovulation, 7
minerals and trace elements, 23–5
  cadmium, mercury, lead, 24–5
  iodine, 23
  iron, 23
  zinc, 23–4
morning sickness, 74

neural tube defects (spina bifida), 25
nutrients, essential, 21
nutrition, 17–26
  in early pregnancy, 18–19
  food deprivation, 17–18
    Dutch Hunger Winter, 18;
    siege of Leningrad, 17
  ideal height and weight, 19

obstetrics experience, previous, 63–8
  miscarriage, 63–6
    causes of, 64; preventing, 65
  previous abnormal deliveries, 68
  previous infant loss, 67–8
  tubal or ectopic pregnancy, 66–7
oestrogen, 8
  test, 53

orgasm, difficulties in attaining, 70
ovulation, 5
  and menstruation, 7
  temperature chart demonstrating, 51

paternal drinking, effects of, 32
perinatal mortality rate, 2
physical factors in sexual problems, 71
the pill, 13–16
  combined, 13–14
  progesterone-only, 15
postcoital test, 53
preconception clinic, 3–4
pregnancy:
  and alcohol abuse, 31–2
  early weeks, 73–5
  and infections, 40–4
    herpes, 43; rubella, 40–3
  tubal or ectopic, 66–7
pregnant mother, and smoking, 28–9
prematurity, 2
prenatal diagnosis, 60–2
  amniocentesis, 61
  chorionic villus sampling, 61
  fetoscopy, 61–2
  ultrasound scans, 60–1
progesterone, 8
  -only pill, 15
  test, 52
prolactin test, 52
proteins, 20
psychological factors in sexual problems, 71

Quetelet index, 19

radiation, ionizing, 3
reproduction, 5–12
  conception, 9–11
  menstrual cycle, 5–8
  sperm production, 9
Royal College of General Practitioners' survey, 14
rubella, 40–3

# *Index*

prevention, 42–3
risk to fetus, 41
status test, 52

semen, 9
  analysis, 50
sex, determination of baby's, 58
sexual problems, 69–72
  affecting females, 70–1
    dyspareunia, 70–1; impaired arousal, 70; libido, 70; orgasms, 70; vaginismus, 70
  affecting men, 69–70
    ejaculation, 69–70; impotence, 69; libido, 69
  causes of, 71
  treatment for, 71–2
smoking, effects of, 27–9
  adverse effects on health, 27–8
  on men, 29
  on pregnant mother, 28–9
  on unborn baby, 29
sperm production, 9
spina bifida, 25
supplementation, in diet, 25–6
  and neural tube defects, 25
surgery, tubal, 54

tetracyclines, 36
thalidomide, 33–5
  history of tragedy, 34–5
thyroid disorders, 46
thyroid gland function test, 52
thyroxine, 46
tobacco, 27–32
  smoking and health, 27–8
toxoplasmosis, 44
tubal pregnancy, predisposing factors, 66–7
tubal surgery, for infertility, 54

ultrasound scans, 60–1
unborn baby, and smoking, 29

vaccinations, against rubella, 42
vaginismus, 70
vitamins, 21–3
  A, 21–2
    deficiency, 25
    B complex, 22
    C, D, 22

warfarin, 36

zinc, 23–4